FOR WHAT IT'S WORTH

A PERSPECTIVE ON HOW TO THRIVE AND SURVIVE PARENTING

AGES 0-2

'Dr. Cook's candid and humorous descriptions of key aspects of raising infants provide a rich, non-formulaic framework for parenting. She succeeds admirably in reflecting on her own feelings, experiences, and thoughts in a way that stimulates each of us to consider our own "best practices" for nurturing emotionally intelligent and hardy children.'

Peter A. Reiner, PhD, LMFT

Licensed Clinical Psychologist/Licensed Marriage and Family Therapist
Faculty at The Feinberg School of Medicine at Northwestern University and
The Chicago Center for Psychoanalysis

Mirador Publishing
10 Greenbrook Terrace
Taunton
Somerset
TA1 1UT

For What It's Worth

*A Perspective on How to Thrive and Survive Parenting
Ages 0-2*

By: Bethany L. Cook, PsyD, MT-BC

DEDICATION

For my two most precious little people, may you continue to grow into your truest selves.

For the Yin of my Yang, none of this would have been possible without you... today and forever you have my heart.

AUTHOR'S NOTES

AT THE AGE OF 37 I quit my job to become a stay-at-home parent. I was completely surprised and caught off-guard at just how unprepared I felt everyday as the challenges of the practical application of full-time parenthood began to overwhelm me.

As a way to cope with these feelings of inadequacy, I began jotting down notes about my experiences because I felt I couldn't be the only parent out there experiencing these feelings. During an especially trying week with my colicky 3 month old, I recalled a young teenage girl I had worked with from Chicago's west-side ghetto.

This young girl was fourteen years old and referred to me by the Courts for therapy because she held her 3-month-old baby upside-down out of a 2-story window. She threatened to drop her small child when the baby's father said he wanted to break up with her.

I reflected on our work together and how she was raised in a family system of abuse and poverty. At the time, I thought to myself there is no way this young woman (or her baby) will ever truly have a chance to break out of this cycle.

However, I firmly believe people *can* and *do* change. One way to make change happen is through education and learning. That scared little 14-year-old girl was always in the back of my mind as I wrote this book. This book had to be relatable, readable and understandable to *all* parents regardless of age, race, educational background or financial means.

Parents of babies and young toddlers have limited time and mental capacity for anything new as they are usually feeling overwhelmed and underwater. Consequently, I worked very hard to make each chapter in this book as short, concise, rich in research and filled with as many funny stories as possible. I chose to add my bibliography at the end of the book because I want you to feel like we are having a conversation between friends, not receiving a lecture from a professor.

This book is for those who want to learn about parenting and/or are excitedly and anxiously awaiting the arrival of the newest family member. I hope my journey helps you with yours.

CONTENTS

SECTION III – Last but NOT Least

SECTION I

Before Baby Arrives

Chapter 1

IN THE BEGINNING
Why Do You Want to Be a Parent?

FOR AS LONG AS I could remember I knew I wanted to be a mom. However, I'm not sure why. What I mean to say is that I am unable to separate the idea of motherhood from what I personally wanted to do with my life. From a young age every decision I have made about my life and educational choices has been geared to blend nicely with the role of mother. I even specialized in working with families and children, for goodness' sake.

When I was little, I thought women didn't have a choice about being a mother, *especially* if she was married. Television shows, movies, magazines and even religion all supported the idea that women essentially had two paths they could take in life: be a sexy, childless, often cold career woman; or a kind, caring, funny, often frumpy and not-so-bright mother. These ideas about who or what a woman should be were also supported by the toys society encouraged my friends and I to play with such as dolls, pretend kitchens, princess dress-up and jewelry making, to name a few.

I was born in 1976 so the toys I grew up with were those from the 1980s: Barbie was queen and Cabbage Patch kids ruled the world. The idea of gender-neutral toys didn't really exist during this time. Even *before* toys began to be commercially manufactured, women were taught and encouraged to take on the nurturing role of mother. My grandmother, who grew up on a farm during the Depression, used to tell me how she made her dolls out of cornhusks. Don't get me wrong, I understand the historical and sociological need for the women of our past to be encouraged to procreate and then care for and nurture their children, but I think we've come along far enough in our developed society that we need to take a step back from this idea and shift our perspective to one that encourages women to embrace what they are naturally inclined to do or to be.

History is full of stories about women who knew their life was designed for something other than motherhood. These brave women were often scorned, ridiculed and even killed because they chose a life that didn't include children. We needn't look any further than Joan of Arc. At age 16 she took a vow of chastity and led the French army to a historical victory over England. She was then captured, tried and convicted for witchcraft and heresy. In 1431 she was killed at the age of 19. Obviously, today's Western society isn't going to kill you if you don't have a baby or choose a different path in life than parenthood. However, I do believe that currently women (and some men), who don't have children are made to feel "less than" those who do have kids. This can be seen in the many microaggressions toward this group of individuals.

A microaggression is an everyday verbal or nonverbal environmental slight, snub, or insult (intentional or not) that communicates hostile, derogatory, or negative messages to a person based solely upon their marginalized group membership, i.e. childless women. An example that fits both men and women who choose to not have children is maternity and paternity leave. What I want to point out is the microaggression toward the men and women who are childless. Employees who don't have kids are seldom if ever offered an equal amount of time off for endeavors that are, to them, of equal value. The United States is definitely behind other developed countries who offer it to parents of newborn children, but that is a rant for another time.

Over and over again I hear stories from mothers and fathers who succumbed to the pressure from a spouse, society, or both and went ahead and had children even though they knew they didn't really want them. These parents aren't necessarily miserable, but they were thrown into a job/role they didn't want. A few of these parents said they were glad that they ended up having children, but others have said they felt their lives would have been fuller if they had lived their truest path.

* ~ * ~ *

When I was 6 years old my parents decided to become members of the Church of Jesus Christ of Latter-Day Saints. I was essentially "raised" Mormon in a small Indiana town. The church had a long list of "do nots" (such as NO premarital sex, NO caffeine, NO drugs, etc.) and I was very loyal to that "list". It was my vision to marry a good Mormon boy and have 5 children, continue to live in the Midwest and fulfill the "dreams of my parents", as they say. But there was one *huge* catch: the church had never definitively told me to *NOT* kiss a girl. (I used to live in a world of black and white, yet, I now know the world is grey… many many shades of grey… *waaaaay* more than 50.) Consequently, the vision of how I would create a family with my partner after marriage was very different from how it actually came to be.

When I met my current life partner/parent partner, it was love at first sight. In many ways she checked all the "traditional" boxes I had created in my head as a child for who I would marry and build a family with, except she didn't have a penis. (I say partner instead of the terms wife/husband/father/mother to define parents in this book because, let's face it… today families are created in many different ways with diverse heads of household: like two dads, two moms, one dad, grandparents, etc.) Anyway, without a penis we would have to start our family in a non-traditional manner. We had two options: 1. adopt, or 2. artificial insemination (AI). Obviously, many heterosexual couples have gone through the adoption/AI route, but this is usually after months/years of trying to get pregnant the old-fashioned way.

The necessity of being non-traditional in starting our family didn't bother me in the slightest. Being and feeling different was something I've always embraced as a way to cope with being, well, a bit odd. For as long as I can remember my mother would always tell me, "You are different and special, Bethany, because you're adopted; that means I wanted you." She told me of how I had lived with my biological mother, grandmother, aunt, had 7 foster parents, was adopted once and returned, and then came to be permanently adopted by my mom and dad at the age of 9 months old. So, starting our family in a non-traditional manner didn't feel odd at all to me.

After a lot of discussion and thought, my partner and I decided we would try the path of artificial insemination. I don't know anything about my biological family's medical history but I have always been strong and healthy. I've never met my biological parents, nor do I know if I have any siblings or half-siblings wandering around and I really wanted to have a genetic connection to another person in this world.

Those reasons, coupled with the fact that my partner's family has a history of unusual and unique health issues, helped with the "who will carry the babies?" decision. I would carry the children and use my own eggs. (*I'll explain more about this in chapter 3*).

I share this story because I strongly believe in the power and need of self-reflection (for some this book may be thinking ahead). Research in psychology shows that self-focus/self-reflection is a critical component to change. Change is inevitable once a new baby comes into your life. To be the best parent you can be requires you to not only look to the future but also reflect a little on the past.

I love my parents very much but knew that there were things they did as a parent that I did not want to do with my children. My parenting goal is to raise healthy, happy, productive humans who will positively contribute to society. As a psychologist, I know that to achieve your goals two things are required. Not only do you need a goal/destination, but you also need the self-awareness of where you currently are (on the metaphorical map) in order to accurately assess the distance between the two. At the end of the day, we cannot reach our targets without knowledge of our current location.

This may be the only parenting book you will read wherein the author, moi, is telling you how challenging parenting can be and how some women and men really loathe it and regret it. Don't stress, there are many, *many* people who enjoy being parents who *also* believe the good outweighs the bad when it comes to being a parent. I am one of them.

Chapter 2

PARENT PARTNER
Pick a Plum

DID YOUR PARENTS EVER talk about the kind of person you should date/marry? Mine did. My mother had two classic lines: 1. *marry a geek, they usually always make good money* 2. *it's just as easy to fall in love with somebody rich as it is to fall in love with somebody poor.* Many will agree that's solid advice; some may not.

Either way, if you consider Dr. Maslow's *Hierarchy of Needs* theory, you will discover that safety is the second most important thing an individual needs to survive. This doesn't mean just a roof over your head, but financial security as well. I did hear the gist of what my mother was saying to me, but instead of looking for a partner to bring home a paycheck, I got myself an education so that I could bring home my own paycheck.

My dad's advice was simply complex. Essentially, he didn't care if I married a person of a different culture or color. His concern was that I married a person who had similar beliefs and came from a similar background to me because, "It will make things easier." I hear where he is coming from; it does make home life run more smoothly if the team is on the same page. Nevertheless, it's unrealistic to think all the pages will align with someone else.

Remember, I have been planning on being a mother and I'm naturally competitive, so consequently I was planning on being the best parent ever. If you're playing a team sport (i.e. family) the way to ensure you *win* is to have not only amazing individual players, but also amazing *team* players.

I knew I wasn't going to settle for just anyone, and I knew my personality wasn't everyone's cup of tea. Consequently, I never turned down a date because "you never know." Maybe this 6 foot 9 inch tall Mormon from Tonga just might be the one!

What I discovered after dating boys and girls from at least 10 different countries and backgrounds was that I didn't mind being single. Another classic one liner from my mother is, "It's better to be single than to wish you were." I definitely agreed with her on that one.

When I finally found my partner at 28, I knew she was the one from the moment I laid eyes on her. The connection was instant for both of us. Of course, her gender wasn't quite what I had been planning on which meant the predetermined "roles" for parenthood were going to be different for us.

She comes from a sports background in tennis and field hockey, and I come from a sports background as well as a music background; at the age of 10 years old I started playing my violin in orchestras and ensembles. We both knew the importance of teamwork, and as parents we had to be a unified front.

Given the fact that her education and career background is finance and accounting whereas mine is psychology and music therapy, we decided I would be the one to put my career on hold and stay home with the kids while they were young. In today's competitive market people "age out" of certain careers and jobs. However, psychology is not one of those fields.

I had always planned on staying home with my children if it was at all possible. My partner and I came to our final conclusion by examining our feelings about two specific markers. 1. How much money would we really be making after we paid either a nanny or daycare? 2. Would the amount of "extra" money earned from my job outweigh the benefits for the children, and family unit, of one parent staying home?

Both research and my experience suggest that families with young babies tend to function the smoothest when one parent is designated "in charge" of the children and/or the running of the house (which means quitting their formal job). That's not to say that homes with two working parents don't run smoothly. It's just feedback from peers/friends/clients/studies that say when one person is in charge of the children/home the family unit has fewer hiccups. It does come at a cost though, and usually to the person staying home, especially if they come from a working background. Their self-esteem and mental health are often areas that suffer as they adjust.

The non-stay-at-home parent is usually the primary money earner and *assists* in duties of child tending and toilet scrubbing. To be honest, sometimes the menial tasks like sweeping and cleaning fall to the parent who is home more, simply because, well, they are home more and therefore may have more opportunity to tidy up. What I learned from waiting tables over the years is this: if you've got time to lean, you've got time to clean.

The distribution of chores/children duties between partners is always something that should be discussed beforehand if possible. Otherwise, resentment quickly builds up about how much you feel like you're doing and they're not doing.

My partner worked 12-13 hour days before we met due to her choice of career and specific job, and she enjoys what she does even though the days are long. She now works 10-12 hour days. She makes sacrifices at the office to spend more time at home. Nevertheless, she just isn't physically around enough for me to say she literally does half the housework.

An important yet less talked about job which usually falls onto the primary parent is what's termed "mental load". The primary parent is usually the one whose brain is constantly juggling things like making plans/appointments, who notices when essentials are running low, who anticipates the emotional and physical needs of the baby(ies), who researches to find/do the best by their family. Essentially, it's like having a lot of apps open on your smartphone, quietly running in the background, silently draining your battery, low… and we're talking "3% left" low.

Unfortunately, the mental load is not just one job, but it is pervasive and applies to nearly all aspects of raising kids and managing a household. To break down mental loads the person carrying them needs to share them with their partner. Sounds easy, right?

I'm sure we've all heard something to the tune of, "Oh, so-and-so is such a great partner. Anytime I need anything done I just ask them and they do it." Great, they do it when asked, but what *I'm* talking about is the fact that the partner has to be *told* and doesn't see it, or naturally think about it on their own. Mental load = mucho energy = draining.

Having a real and honest conversation with your partner about these "non-visual" mental apps running in your background is very important. Maybe it is impractical for your partner to literally do half of everything but find a few things they can realistically do and let them.

For example, my partner is responsible for setting up/reminding me about dog-related things such as vet appointments and giving them their monthly worming pills. She is also in charge of making sure all the monthly bills are paid on time, among other things.

Often, I hear the primary parent say things like, "It's just easier if I do it because they (partner) will mess it up anyway." They definitely won't do things exactly like you do but you have to give them a chance to try and share the mental burden of everything that is constantly running in the background when managing a home and young children (and in my case, two dogs, too).

In my very feminist household, I decided while the children are young that I would don the dress of domestic goddess and essentially become a 1950's housewife. Actually, I do NOT wear a dress, it's more like baggy, paint stained sweatpants and the cleanest-smelling top I can find.

This is *my* choice and I am doing it out of love for both of my children and my partner. I believe in the importance and benefits of having one parent stay home full-time with young children. Plus, I don't do *everything* a 1950's housewife was supposed to do; my partner has to cope with a glass of wine instead of a freshly mixed cocktail when she gets in from work at 8:30 PM.

All jokes aside, being a full-time stay at home parent is the hardest, *the* hardest job I've ever had, and let me tell ya, I've had my share of interesting and sometimes gross jobs. And from what I hear from other parents who stay home, and even those who work outside the home, staying home full-time with a baby/babies/toddlers is the hardest thing they've ever done. Some of my friends even confided they *couldn't* stay home with their young children 24/7 because they would go nuts. Bravo to them for knowing their limits.

While not all parents/couples have the option to have one parent stay home full-time with their babies, there are many parents in a position financially, with budgeting, that could have one person stay home but they still choose to work. That's JUST HOW BLOODY HARD IT IS! So let's, as a society, start giving more props to the women *and* men who stay home with their children instead of making them feel like "it's not enough to *just* be a stay-at-home parent".

Not only do you and your partner have to cope with all the changes and additional responsibilities that come with children, but you will both need to be understanding of the growth and personal changes each of you will go through when you go from being a "cool chick" to a mother, or from being a "dank, dope dude" to being a dad.

Going from a "couple" to the "couple with a new baby" is also a transition. Be patient with each other during this time and know that your babies won't be young forever, and eventually you will get more time with your partner again and begin to feel like a couple again. Remember, neither of you will be getting the same amount of sleep you once did. Be warned and be prepared. You both have no clue who you may become once you've been sleep deprived (on any level) for a few months.

If you are a single parent or your partner travels, you will have to seek other people in your life to help out. My partner sometimes needs to travel for work and during the first year of life as the "couple with a new baby" she was gone for a cumulative total of 60 days due to her mother's failing health. My family lives around 2 hours away, which meant they could help out on occasion but not as much as was needed.

Consequently, during the first year with my oldest child I was home alone with a newborn for stretches of a week at a time and sought help from neighbors. I invited him and myself to their houses in the evenings. I'm not sure they had much choice in the matter, but hey, I needed a break, lucky them. Also, I was blessed to have a neighbor (she literally lives across the street), who, from the first day we brought our son home, lovingly volunteered her time to help us. She had raised 4 boys, knew the ropes and just how hard it was and she wanted to pay it forward. I wouldn't have survived without her help and support.

Often it is difficult for new parents to admit they need help for fear that others will think they are failures as parents. The way I was able to cope with these negative feelings was to remind myself that I was not alone in my struggle. Also, shifting my perspective helped. I reminded myself that history has shown us time and time again, that survival of the species demands we humans cooperate and work as a cohesive group.

It's only in recent history that the need to live close to your family for survival and support has declined. I'm sure there are small towns in the world that still have the village community feeling, but for the most part parents are forced to create their village with people near and far that they can rely on to help with the rearing of their children. Some of these people will be paid and some won't.

Be picky about the people you let into your village. Just because someone is family doesn't mean they automatically get to babysit. Just because someone is family doesn't mean they will agree with the ways you parent and may disregard your rules. Sometimes it might be easier on the children to pay someone to watch the kids so you know that they will listen (hopefully) to what you want rather than asking family who are free but don't respect the boundaries you set for your kid(s).

Yet again, many people don't have the extra cash to pay someone else to watch their children, so family members/close friends do. It's a huge plus if your family is close and all work together nicely and they respect your style of parenting. But it's a huge pain in the bum if your extended family doesn't respect your choices and ignores your requests when they are around your children.

It takes a village to raise a child. Get as many people whom you trust and whose opinions and outlook on parenting you value into your close circle of friends. If you want to try and work with difficult family members, great! If you would rather limit your children's exposure to people who are toxic (friends and/or family) then do it! Just make sure you seek out and find people who cherish and respect you and your child.

Chapter 3

NON-TRADITIONAL BABY MAKING
IVF and IUI

FOR THOSE WHO HAVE been through it before, for those who have thought about it but didn't need to go through it, and for the rest of you who haven't a bloody clue how two chicks make a baby, I'm gonna break it down for you. (Keep in mind some couples don't just need to find sperm to complete their family but also an egg and potentially a surrogate to carry the embryo.)

Before scientific breakthroughs in artificial insemination, people who wanted a child had two choices. They could have heterosexual sex and hope they get pregnant or adopt a child. Whilst those options are still available today, many couples, gay or straight, are physically unable to have a child together. Nevertheless, science now makes the possibility a bit easier even though there still isn't a 100% guarantee of getting pregnant using science.

My partner and I were fortunate that we just needed sperm to get our family started. After much discussion we decided to go with an anonymous donor and use an online donor bank to find our donor dad. (Please note that every family will have their own terms for how they refer to individuals whose DNA helped create their children/family.)

I absolutely LOVED searching through a catalog of men/sperm donors looking for the "perfect stud" whilst my partner did not. So it was decided that I would narrow down potential donors and she would approve the final cut.

We wanted someone who shared as many physical, intellectual and temperament/personality characteristics as my partner: and each donor bank has varying degrees of information about donor dad/mom. Of course, no one could be a perfect match and questions like "Do I choose the guy who has the right color hair and eyes or the one whose temperament/personality is a match?" often come into play. Knowing what I know about humans and their behavior made us focus more on the donor's temperament and personality rather than just his looks.

We were fortunate though because we just happened to find a man who has the same temperament as my partner. According to the Keirsey Temperament Sorter report only 8% of the world shares his and my partner's personality characteristics. Our donor also shared many of my partner's physical characteristics. What luck!

Once we found the sperm, the next big step involved the practical aspects of getting the egg and sperm to meet. First, let me say that if you're stressed out for any reason, the likelihood that you will get pregnant decreases significantly; it doesn't matter how you try to get pregnant, keep stress to a minimum.

That being said, when I first met with my gynecologist I was stressed out. Not only was I focusing a lot of my energy trying hard to get my mind and body ready to get pregnant, I was working full-time doing neuropsychological assessments, driving a reverse commute from the Northside of Chicago to a southwest suburb, and my doctor's office was located downtown Chicago. Who cares where my doctor's office is, right? WRONG! This is the place where the not-so-private act of having a person in a lab coat squirt some sperm up your crotch happens, mate. Not a pretty picture, I know, and I'm sorry. I'm sure there are others, who choose to try and inseminate at home, maybe with incense, candles, and romantic music playing in the background, but I'm not a patient person and I wanted to take the most direct and potentially successful route.

I shared my experience because I wanted you to get a nice in-your-face feel for just how *un*romantic, sterile and stressful getting pregnant this way can be. (I know plenty of straight couples who have said that baby making sex becomes pretty mechanical and unromantic as well.) I'm getting ahead of myself though. Before insemination is attempted many women start taking hormone drugs. I'm gonna say it again slowly just in case you missed what I said… h o r m o n e *drugs*!

Anyone who has taken IUI or IVF drugs (I'll explain exactly what these letters mean in just a second) knows one thing for sure… THEY MAKE YOU CRAZY! No joke, after a few months of an on-again off-again regimen of hormone drugs, a person can quickly and easily become a "hot mess". For example, I was walking down a neighborhood street and a person looked at me in a manner that I perceived as negative and I almost punched them in the face. I raced home to tell my partner because I was so freaked out by my unusual reaction.

So, what are all these acronyms and what do they mean? Intrauterine insemination (IUI) is a fertility treatment that involves placing sperm inside a woman's uterus to facilitate fertilization. The goal of IUI is to increase the number of sperm that reach the fallopian tubes and subsequently increase the chance of fertilization (think turkey baster scenes from movies).

Because IUI is less invasive, we went this route first. Nevertheless, I still had to take hormone drugs and get regular ultrasounds to see if I had any good-looking follicles (eggs). If everything looked good, then my partner (who loved this part), had to give me a shot in the ass with more hormones to make sure my egg released from the ovary and was heading down the fallopian tube to meet up with some sperm.

Then 2-4 days later I would go back to the doctor's office where he would shoot in the sperm. We did this dance 3 times over the course of 8 months. Why 8 months? Well, some months the eggs didn't look great, or I was out of town, or my period didn't line up with timing and work, etc. Although stressful and time consuming to say the least, I was lucky that my boss was understanding and gave me extra time to make all these appointments.

Many bosses, both male and female, show no compassion or understanding toward people trying to get pregnant in a non-traditional way. And on a related side note… during the early 2000s I was at my music therapy internship and I overheard a physician tell another employee that "…she is gonna get pregnant again anyway so maybe we can just eliminate her position before she returns. She's costing us lots of money every time she takes maternity leave."

No, I didn't say anything to anyone because I didn't know who they were referencing and at that time in my life I didn't feel empowered enough as a woman to say anything to this physician. However, if I heard him say this today, I definitely would confront him. Nevertheless, these are the types of microaggressions that I am referring to when it comes to how the media, public leaders, and off-handed comments impact how both men and women feel about themselves with regard to parenthood. Okay, off of my side note.

Yet regardless of all the drugs, attempts, and ultrasounds, 8 months later I still wasn't pregnant. Acupuncture was even attempted to help increase my fertility. I think the most frustrating part was not knowing if the sperm/egg were meeting… was there something wrong with me, with the egg/fallopian tubes/uterus/sperm, etc.? All these "unknowns" needed to be explored and addressed so we could brace ourselves for how we should move forward, such as: "Yeah, everything is working so it's just a matter of time," or "Nope, your ovaries aren't functioning properly so you're going to need medical intervention," or "You're not going to be able to get pregnant so maybe you should think about adoption."

Enter IVF. The formal definition of in vitro fertilization (IVF) is a complex series of procedures used to treat fertility or genetic problems and assist with the conception of a child. During IVF, mature eggs are collected (retrieved) from a woman's ovaries following hormone treatment and fertilized with sperm in a lab. My version is a little less medical and gives you a little more "feel" for what it was like.

I took tons and tons of different pills like birth control (physicians do this so they can regulate and control your menstrual cycle), gave myself daily shots of hormones around my belly button and even had the pleasure of inserting progesterone pills into my vagina twice a day for 2 weeks after the transfer of the embryo. Let's just say it's not a walk in the park for anyone involved; my mood swings and hot flashes were enough to strain my otherwise strong relationship with my partner and those closest to me.

As I mentioned already, I am not a patient person and by the time we looked into IVF we had been "trying" to get pregnant for about 8 months. Being impatient does not help anyone when trying to get pregnant and neither does being competitive. I knew very little about IVF when I started the process, but what I had heard was that when taking these types of hormone drugs women often release many eggs (like 20). So, when my competitive side learned that I only had 10 eggs I felt like a failure as a woman. My awesome physician kept saying it didn't matter how many eggs, what mattered was their quality. His words helped me a little bit, but I still felt like a failure.

My first IVF didn't work. The physician was "shocked" because the embryo was "perfect." Nevertheless, on the second IVF attempt a few months later, it worked and Arthur was born in late July.

Nineteen months later Ivy came to us via IUI (remember turkey baster method). Out of the blue Arthur decided he was done breastfeeding, just like that, and refused the boob when he was 10 months old. My partner and I were trying to time the space between the children to be around 24 months. We were getting ready to visit family in the UK and I knew how much was involved in getting pregnant via IVF, so I went to my physician to just "check-in" before we took off and to get ready to start the birth control regime so we could get my period timed up for the IVF track.

Yet, when I went to the physician to have a routine check-up before we started the IVF process they noticed I had a "perfect" follicle ready to drop so I jokingly told my partner we should just "send in the sperm" to save me the pain of all the IVF requirements. The speed at which she agreed makes me believe she was *not* looking forward to the hormone ride from hell she experienced last time with me and was more than happy to oblige the IUI route. Lo and behold, it worked. Consequently, the kids came 19 months apart, not 24 months, and my life changed much faster than I anticipated.

Chapter 4

BIRTH

It's Nothing Like the Movies

AT 5:00 AM ON A HOT summer morning, I slowly dragged my 9-month pregnant and sweaty bum out of bed and shuffled off to the bathroom for what was the millionth pee that night. I sat on the loo with my eyes closed I was so tired, finished my business, stood up and as warm water ran down my leg I thought, "What is going on? I just peed!"

And before I could have another sleepy thought, more liquid started trickling down my leg, a mild trickle, not tons, but enough to be uncomfortable and noticeable. I yelled to my partner, half awake, to, "Come here, I think I keep peeing uncontrollably on the floor!" My partner raced to the bathroom, took one look and said, "Uh, I think your water broke." Duh, did I feel like an idiot. I guess I was expecting the massive gush we see on TV followed by mere seconds before the baby is born, right?

Once your water breaks it's not just a "one time" trickle, fluid continues to periodically flow down your legs. I didn't know this, I don't remember anyone telling me this, but I quickly learned that I didn't know as much as I thought I did about giving birth even though I believed I had done my research.

Birth for me was NOTHING like I had seen in the movies or the stories I had heard from other people. This was my first birth and I read that it's rare for a woman's water to break naturally but even more so for the first-born.

The fact that my water broke didn't mean my baby was coming anytime soon. In fact, my partner, our doula (a trained professional who provides continuous physical, emotional and informational support to a mother before, during and shortly after childbirth) and I hung around in the hospital room "waiting" for labor to kick-in for 7 hours.

During those 7 hours my contractions didn't feel strong and I laughed and said, "This is gonna be easy if this is all it is." I should have kept my motormouth shut because right at the 7-hour mark the physician came in and suggested we start Pitocin to get the labor moving. Pitocin is the synthetic version of oxytocin, the natural hormone that helps your uterus contract during labor. I spoke to my partner and we decided to go ahead with the Pitocin.

I had really wanted to have as natural a birth as I could. I would have done it at home in a blow-up pool if my partner had been cool with it. She is warier of the potential risks and the importance of having medical teams close for the "just in case" moments so the thought of a home birth did not sit well with her. Since I was fine having a baby in a hospital, that's what we did.

Often new mothers/parents are asked to make a birth plan. A birth plan is a way for you to communicate your wishes to your birth team who are the ones who care for you during labor. You don't have to write one up, but at least check out what types of questions a template birth plan asks and make sure you're ready with answers when the time comes. Things can quickly go from good to bad, and a birth plan tells your birth team about the type of labor and birth you'd like to have, what you want to happen, and what you want to avoid.

My partner and I had a neatly typed up birth plan with us and on this plan it stated I did NOT want an epidural, unless I reeeeeaaallly *reeeeeaaallly* needed it. Remember a few paragraphs ago when I mentioned I didn't know everything about birth even though I had read everything I could find? Well, I didn't know that once a woman is given Pitocin that her body starts to have continuous contractions. That means there are no "breathing breaks" where you can catch your breath and the pain subsides. Instead your uterus continually tries to rip itself apart forcing a watermelon out of a small stretchy hole the size of a lemon.

Since I didn't realize I was going to have continuous contractions, and I desperately wanted to see how "tough" I was without an epidural, I endured 7 hours straight of contractions. Seven hours of constant pain like I had never experienced. I wanted to spend the entire time in the shower. Baths were only provided for the women who used midwives instead of physicians. Every room should have a place for the mom to float in because the hot water felt AMAZING on my aching body for those 7 hours. To get my hot water fix I was forced to try and find a comfortable position at the bottom of a shower as the streaming water pounded on my sore and tired back.

I paced the room, I cussed a lot, and tried hard, oh so hard to work through the pain. I kept saying, "I just need a 60 second break," in between strings of profanities. I was butt-ass naked because even wearing a hospital gown annoyed me. Every time the gown touched my skin it felt like a cross between fire and a tickle. I also had an annoying medical drip cart attached to me as I crawled in and out of the shower and on and off the bed trying to find a comfortable position.

Finally, after a total of 14 hours of labor, I sat on the edge of the bed and quietly, gently and politely said to my partner and doula, "I'm done; please may I have an epidural?" Immediately startled and stunned by my obvious change in tone, the lack of the cuss words and use of manners, both my partner and doula knew that I was dead serious.

The pain was so intense that I was petrified I wasn't going to be able to sit still and the epidural needle would puncture my spine and I would be paralyzed. Yes, I remember I said I didn't want to have an epidural, but like I also said: go in with a plan but be open to change.

Luckily the needle went in smoothly and I just sat back and waited for the effects to set-in. The staff simply told me to change the side I was laying on occasionally so the drugs would be dispersed evenly throughout my body. That seemed easy to do, but when I turned over to my left side 5 minutes later baby Arthur's heart rate dropped. Apparently, the umbilical cord was wrapped around his neck in such a way that when I lay on my left side it cut off his blood flow. The long and the short of this story is that only half of my body was numb for the birth of Arthur. But eh, whatta ya gonna do?

After 21 hours of labor, Arthur was born in three pushes. No, really. The doctor came in and said it looked like we were ready to push so she told me to, "Give it a go." Arthur came out so quickly she wasn't able to get the "oops-if-I-drop-the-baby-this-table-will-catch-it" table ready and she literally caught him. He was born to the song *Come What May* from *Moulin Rouge*. I made a massive mix of songs I love which we played throughout labor/birth, and it was like Russian roulette to see which song he would be born to.

When Ivy was born, 19 months later, I was in pre-labor with her for 24 hours *before* any real action started. My water didn't break, and because everything you read says that the second child comes much more quickly than the first, my partner and I started to become concerned after 16 hours of mild contractions with the timing in between them ranging from 10-15 minutes. My partner, doula and I even went to the hospital only to be told I was dilated around 2-3 cm. I was advised to walk circles around the corridor for 2 hours to see if that "helped move things along." All that walking did was chafe my inner thighs in a hospital gown that didn't cover my enormous pregnant body.

Plus, I was struggling with feeling stupid that I didn't even know my body well enough to know if I was going into active labor or not. Man, I was so hard on myself during those 2 hours of walking. To distract myself from my thoughts I chatted with my doula about her children.

The walking did nothing to move labor along and we drove home at 3:30 AM. I couldn't sleep due to the continual contractions that were still coming but just weren't going anywhere in intensity until 1:00 PM the next day. My contractions started slowly increasing in intensity and duration, but it wasn't until 7:00 PM in the evening (24 hours after they started) that my contractions were strong enough for me to go back to the hospital. I had just finished cooking some chicken tortilla soup and I was definitely going to have at least one bowl before leaving for the hospital. (The physicians recommended not eating after I went into labor. I didn't eat before Arthur but I was definitely gonna have a bowl of soup before we headed downtown to the hospital to deliver Ivy.)

By the time we got to the hospital I was dilated to around 6/7cm. The goal is 10cm and a lot of pushing and more pain before a birth can happen. I thought I had felt enough pain at 7cm and asked for an epidural. Two doctors came in; one was a resident in training. Again, I sat very very still but became quite annoyed with the banter the boys at my back were making. The hospital policy is that everyone leaves the room except the doctor giving the epidural, so my partner and nurse didn't overhear their conversation, which went something like this. But keep in mind I was mid-labor here.

Resident: *There is a lady in 231 that is requesting an epidural.*

Doctor: *Yeah, I saw that. I know this lady. She has had like 4 kids and is already dilated to 8 cm. Don't know why she needs one now, she knows how it feels to give birth and she's almost there anyway.*

Resident: *Okay, well, what do I do? Shall I go there now?*

Doctor: *Yeah, go check on her and see if you can change her mind, I wanna take a break.*

Resident: *Okay.*

During this awesome bedside banter the resident had attempted to insert the needle *twice*, each time not getting it "right". They asked me once during this conversation if I was "okay". Like what was I gonna say? "Your bedside chitchat is making me mad and nervous and if this f*cking resident doesn't get the needle in right this time, ya'll can go f*ck yourself!" But I just said, "Yup," breathing through the pain and anger. The resident comes back.

Resident: *I spoke to the woman and she is adamant about wanting an epidural.*

Doctor: *Fine. Come watch me so I can finish up here and move on.*

Yes, the doctor was able to successfully insert the needle into my spine and I finally got some relief, both for my body but also my ears. I told my partner as soon as she came back in what had happened. Both she and I were furious but felt we couldn't complain in case of retaliation. You know, like pissing off a waiter and hoping they don't spit in your water. Since we were in a vulnerable place and needed the staff to like us, we kept silent. Looking back, I'm not proud of being silent, but that's what happened.

Unfortunately, I was still feeling intense contractions, so the epidural dose was increased, twice. When the pain was finally manageable, I was so relieved that I sat up quickly and started singing along to a song that was playing on my mix. Then the room began to spin and go dark and all I remember was that the machines started beeping and people started shouting for the nurses. My blood pressure and pulse dropped and so did Ivy's; they laid me back down in the bed and that seemed to settle things down. What I remember the most during this event was that I hoped it wasn't triggering my partner who had recently been by her mother's side as she passed away.

Nothing else very significant happened except when it came time to push, my physician started having a "back and forth" with the head nurse about how and when I needed to push; this of course was confusing to me so I wasn't pushing at all during the contractions which was irritating my physician. My physician ended up telling the nurse to back off, "She's done this before," and in 6 pushes out came Ivy to the song *Rainbow Connection*. She was almost born to *Regulate* by Warren G, which would have fit her personality a bit better. At the end of the day, I had two completely different experiences.

I have heard of women who have short, easy births but I didn't believe those women really existed and that it was just a wives' tale told to pregnant women to help them mentally prepare for birth. Guess what, it is *not* a wives' tale! One of my close friends delivered her second baby in her home on the floor; she told me she was on her hands and knees and saw her son's head crowning. So, she took one of her hands to feel how close he was and ended up catching him in her hands/arms. She is European and had a midwife in her home. From start to finish her entire labor and birth was a total of 2.5 hours. I share this because until she had her second child, I had yet to meet someone who had easy and quick labors/births.

My wrap-up words are these: nothing will ever go exactly as planned, so try to be flexible and just go with the flow. Birth plans are good to have and it's helpful to know what you want in an ideal birth situation. Relax and try to enjoy it if you can.

SECTION II

After Baby Arrives

Chapter 5

BUILD YOUR BABY'S BRAIN THROUGH TOUCH
Your Warm Loving Arms Won't Spoil your Baby

ARTHUR WAS PROBABLY AROUND 2-3 weeks old when one of my grandmas told me that I was going to "spoil him" if I kept responding to every cry/noise of distress he made and by holding him all the time. This wasn't the first time I had heard that holding and trying to calm a crying baby would spoil them. This line of thinking never made sense to me and after all my "book learning" I finally understood why.

The human brain is born with billions of neurons and it is the experience of social interaction and communication that wires the brain to either its full potential or to a "lesser" more compromised state. Ignoring/neglecting your baby means that the brain may not be "fed" enough social interaction to help it grow to its optimal best.

I know that I was neglected for the first 9 months of my life. My parents collected my on a hot summer afternoon. They shared with me that I was sprawled on my back in a playpen right by the open front door of an old farmhouse. I had ear wax coming out of my ears, I was covered in dirt, there was a cow penned up near the front porch and flies were buzzing everywhere. I had small red marks all over my body that my parents thought were either fly bites or chicken pox. Turns out they were fly bites; I had to get the chickenpox vaccine as an adult.

As the story goes my mom said she held me on her lap as car seats weren't that strict back in the day, barely touching me or my clothes on the way home since I was so dirty. The first thing she did with me once we were home was to put me in a bath.

She said I didn't smile or engage with others for several months, and once I started coming out of my "shell" my smiles and happiness was reserved for the men in my life. I had issues with women, thought to be due to the neglect I received from them for the first few months of life.

My mom also shared that the only time I let her hold/comfort me was when I was little and had growing pains in my legs. Other than that, I didn't want affection or comfort from others. I had learned during my first few months of life that my caretakers couldn't be trusted or depended on; I had already developed a general mistrust of the world.

A psychologist named Erik Erikson developed a theory that examines the psychosocial stages of human development. His first stage (0-23 months old), focuses on whether the child's basic needs are met such as food, affection, and receiving comfort when crying; this stage is labeled Trust vs. Mistrust.

If parents are engaged and working hard to meet the demands of their young baby/child then over the first 2 years of their life the child learns to trust their parents and consequently themselves and starts to confidently explore the world around them. It's through these early interactions that our ego develops as we successfully resolve crises that are distinctly social in nature.

The idea of the ego comes from Freud, known as the father of modern day psychology, who believed it (ego), develops to mediate between the Id (natural impulses like the need for immediate gratification) and the external real world. If you don't like the psycho-babble you could think of the ego as that little angel that sits on your shoulder who encourages you to make the right choices and control your naughty/selfish/animalistic impulses. The Id would then be the little devil that sits on your other shoulder and encourages you to act on every one of those impulses and desires.

No, I'm not saying your infant is cognitively capable of metacognition (essentially thinking about thinking), what I'm saying is that by touching and interacting and responding to your baby and their cries you help build a neural foundation that supports a healthy developing ego as well as the neural pathways that will be the foundation for their executive function abilities: impulse control, delaying instant gratification, self-regulation, judgment and reasoning.

A famous study done in 1958 by Harry Harlow involved baby Rhesus monkeys. These monkeys were taken from their mothers and put in a cage with two metal surrogate mothers. One was made out of bare wire: cold and unyielding to the touch. However, this bare wire monkey held the food/bottle for the infant monkey. The other fake monkey mother was also made from wire but covered in soft comfortable material and easy to snuggle into.

What they discovered was that the infant monkey would spend all of its time clinging to the soft monkey and only went to the wire monkey when it needed food. After the baby monkey would eat, it would quickly return to the soft and comforting monkey mother. This study suggested that infant love was not a simple response to the satisfaction of physiological needs being met (feeding), but that an infant *also* needed physical touch and interaction to thrive and survive.

Here's the thing, your baby needs you to respond to them when they communicate with you. Tears and screams are the most effective way for them to tell us they need something. Ironically, parents want to run away from that noise or do anything in their power to stop it. One of the hardest things to accept as a parent is that sometimes we simply can't stop the cries.

Reflecting on both my babies, I couldn't be around them if they were crying and not experience a physiological reaction; the inside of my body would begin to feel this surge of nervous energy and it was uncomfortable. As a result, my desire to reach out, to hold and comfort them every time they cried was greatly influenced by my physical response to the screams.

Once, during a very stressful time when I was completely at my wits' end as to how to get Arthur to stop crying (we were heading toward the second full hour of tears… how I *love* colic which kicks up toward the end of the day), I securely strapped him in a baby bouncer that electronically gently rocked him and left him in the house alone whilst I went out back to the farthest corner of the yard, sat down and stared at the grass, feeling completely numb as tears streamed out of my eyes. I had to go to this extreme to stop the physical pain/energy I was experiencing. I numbly cried at the knowledge that being around my baby made me feel this way.

Knowing what I know about the importance of being "there" for your crying baby only made it harder because I have high expectations for myself and parenting. It was at this point when I had to tell myself that he would be OK crying alone for a few minutes in the house whilst I cried alone outside. If I couldn't hear him cry I didn't have to deal with the physical response of my body.

After I had regrouped, I went back inside. Arthur was still crying but I had calmed myself enough to try to comfort him again. Since I was completely drained of emotional resources, we both went upstairs to the rocking chair and I just held him, patted his back, rocked him and learned how to sit in that uncomfortable space. You know the one where you feel completely helpless and that feeling of helplessness makes you want to act or do something; makes you feel like a complete failure as a parent?

I fought that urge and just sat in the room being present for my infant's pain and tears, and he finally fell asleep after 2 ½ hours of crying. All *I* had to do was to learn how to sit in the uncomfortable space of a crying baby and come to terms with my own feelings of inadequacy and physical discomfort. I made my inner voice keep telling my insecure self that I wasn't inadequate I was trying so very hard, and both he and I were going to survive.

I did survive and so did my babies. Remember, it is these first early relationships that drive brain development. Our babies are primed to be interested in human faces (but prefer the primary caregiver the most), and enjoy initiating non-verbal communication with others by cooing, babbling and my personal favorite: crying.

When we respond to an infant's intense gaze, smiles or babbling we set up a chain of back and forth exchanges that are central to the wiring and sculpting of the brain. The ability of our babies to learn how to regulate their own emotions, behaviors and attention spans increases over time with maturity, experience and most importantly responsive relationships. SO GO TOUCH YOUR BABIES!

Chapter 6

MANY ROADS LEAD TO ROME
Many Ways to Raise a Baby

I WAS INCREDIBLY OVERWHELMED with my first child Arthur and his colic. I found myself poring over research papers, parenting blogs, professional advice, religious advice and anything else I could get my hands on to read. Remember, I was now a full-time stay at home mom… 24/7… every single minute… of every day… having just come out a job which required neuropsychological testing and report writing. I was bored out of my bloody mind and believed that "out there" in the vast world of the Internet, someone had cracked the code about how to stop a baby crying, or how to get a baby to nap for longer than 2 hours, or how to fart a baby when they have wind (yes, it all exists and it can be Googled).

Yet, what I found was there is *NO ONE PERFECT WAY TO RAISE YOUR BABY.* Yes I italicized and capped that sentence and I meant to because it is that important to me for you to recognize and accept that every baby/child is different and the only things out there are "tools" and "options" or "ideas" to help you manage your child's behavior in the least restrictive way possible.

Let me just say during those early months with the children that I spent over 2000+ hours of research on babies and all their lovely "symptoms", like farting, pooing, throwing-up, getting sick, not sleeping, eating issues, breastfeeding, etc. (My heart goes out to parents whose children have additional health and cognitive issues as I know your path is much different from mine and very *very* difficult.) What I found out was that many claimed to have found "the one and only perfect way" to fix this or that.

I'm here to tell you there isn't a one-size-fits-all when it comes to raising kids. Each baby is different and is constantly changing so just when you think you've got their naptime routine down – *wham!* – they start mastering a skill like rolling, or get a cold, and it throws everything out of whack.

Now before you panic too much about the fact that you will never find a quick fix or a cure for all the stresses parenthood brings, take comfort in the knowledge that you get to create the best and most individualized way to raise your child, as long as you're willing to be flexible in your attitude and the techniques you use. When you find yourself at the end of your rope, tie a knot, hold on, and think about how many days old you are and how many days old your child is. Take an objective perspective about the situation and just keep *trying*.

When your baby wants to sleep in your arms and that means you don't get a lot of sleep, then you have to figure out how you're going to cope with the lack of sleep while allowing your baby to sleep. My partner and I both agreed having one person sleep-deprived is better than having two… plus babies usually want their primary caregiver as comfort, so as the genetic and stay-at-home parent, I was "it".

Yes, there were times when I was sick or I needed to sleep a little extra due to deprivation, and my partner would jump in and take over. It wasn't always easy and 99% of the time Ivy refused help/love/cuddles from my partner or anyone other than me, causing both anger and frustration on my end as well as my partner's. To add to the frustration, I was sometimes too tired and emotionally drained to offer comfort to my partner as she cried when our daughter refused to be held by her.

Every parent has a story or two about how they tried one thing with one kid and had to do a totally different approach with another one. As parents, we have to be constantly adapting and changing as well. We learn how to hold in a sneeze just as the baby has *finally* gone to sleep, or we learn how to unwrap a piece of candy or open a bag of chips without a child hearing.

We become ninjas and do it because they need it. We do it because we are older and we do it because we love our babies. As their primary caregivers and providers, we should consistently and without regard, provide hugs, cuddles, lullabies, car rides, and stroller-walks-in-the-middle-of-a-Chicago-blizzard types of commitments to do whatever it takes to make the baby feel happy and stress-free. But don't get me wrong, I'm not saying your child will and should always be the center of your attention and life.

What I am saying is that for at least the first 365 days you've got to suck it up… being a parent totally blows a lot of the time. Your job is to try and gain a perspective of the situations that stress you out with your kid and deal with them for at least 365 days. And remember, there will never be just one way to raise your child or one technique that will always work to get them to eat, or fart, or sleep, or whatever.

The rate at which a baby's brain, body and skill sets develop in the first year is unbelievable. What comes with that rapid development is the need for a safe, stable, comforting and constant foundation of love and support from their parent(s). Put in the work early and you shall reap the benefits later.

Chapter 7

SLEEP LIKE A BABY, OR NOT

Sleep Deprivation and Its Impact on Parents

BEFORE I HAD CHILDREN, I had never been awake for 24 hours straight without sleep. I came close once when my best friend told me, months in advance, that for her 24th birthday I had better mentally prepare because she expected me to party with her all night. At the time, I lived in Chicago and she lived in Southern California and I was heading her way for the week.

As a very competitive person I find it hard to refuse a challenge; needless to say, I stayed awake for 22 hours straight and survived to regale the fun and interesting stories of the shenanigans we got into that night. Even in all my years of higher education (16 years), I never stayed up all night studying or writing a paper. Then, at the ripe age of 37 I had my first child and the world, as I knew it, no longer existed.

I have always loved sleep and require a good 8-9 hours a night if I am to function at my optimal capacity. (Having babies will teach you just how much sleep you need to feel functional and how much you need to merely survive.) Anyway, my body gets tired around 8:30 PM. It just does... I don't know why, I've tried to shift it... sometimes I can push through to 9-9:30 but by then consider me mentally asleep and not responsible for anything agreed to or said during a conversation after 9:00 PM.

Ever since I was a child, I've felt I was fighting for my "sleep space" (sleep space is a term I created which means an allotted amount of time set aside each day for an individual to be in an environment conducive to relaxation and sleep; i.e. bedroom, quiet corner of the house on a couch, moving car, etc.). Again, remember my ideal sleep space is 8-9 hours (and yes, I am one of those lucky people who is usually asleep when my head hits the pillow). If I don't get enough sleep I don't function well, no one does really, and so I've always been pretty strict about my sleep routine and know myself enough to know I am a morning person and need to go to bed at night.

Since my children were born 19 months apart it meant I was never able to "catch up" on sleep in between having babies. I became pregnant when Arthur was 10 months old and I think most women who carried their children would say sleeping while pregnant is difficult in general due to a myriad of reasons including the urge to pee all the time, the sweats, babies kicking, nausea, worry, stress, etc.

From birth, my children were able to sleep for 4-6 hour stretches a night before "needing something" from me, such as a cuddle, food, a diaper change, etc. This lasted until they were around 5 months old and they began mastering the skill of rolling.

Here's the deal: once a baby starts mastering skills like rolling, sitting up, or crawling, it means their sleep will be disrupted because their little brains are so excited about learning new things that sometimes it will wake them at night as they try to continue mastering the task. This translates into horrible sleep for parents as we hold them, rock them, and reassure them we will always be there for them when they need us. This type of support means parents' needs get moved aside.

Guess what? After your baby starts rolling, the teeth start coming around 6-10 months. Arthur's teething was pretty typical. His drool wasn't excessive, and a simple bandana tied around his neck caught the lovely spit.

Then enter Ivy, who got 8 teeth at once when she was 6 months old. It was at this time that my world spiraled out of control because I was getting 1-3 hours of broken sleep a night trying to tend to my crying and uncomfortable baby. (Bear in mind Arthur would still wake on occasion and need a cuddle; most of the time he was OK with my partner comforting him, but as my partner said to me a long time ago, "Sometimes nothing helps but a cuddle from the main momma.") My new and horrific sleeping "pattern" continued for 6 months.

So, you ask, what happens to a person when they are severely sleep-deprived? Great question! Let me break it down for you. Besides becoming a complete and utter jerk to almost everyone around me including the kids, my body, mind and personality underwent many unfortunate changes.

Here is a glance at what happens to a person who is experiencing sleep deprivation. I've not listed everything and the list isn't ranked in any particular order; I just wanted to provide a quick overview of how much can go wrong with a person who is sleep deprived. And I'm talking just being 3-5 hours behind on sleep can cause symptoms. It should be noted that science has shown it is *possible* to catch up on lost sleep if you take a nap or sleep in over the weekend.

Changes That Happen Due to Sleep Deprivation

<u>Body</u>:
◊ Slurred speech
◊ Uncontrolled reflexive movements of the eye (similar to being intoxicated)
◊ Decreased immunity
◊ Slight shakiness or hand tremors
◊ Reduced threshold for seizures
◊ Subtle changes in body temperature, blood pressure, heart rate, breathing rate
◊ Hormone changes which impact weight and thyroid functioning
◊ and in extreme cases, death. YES, DEATH from not sleeping

Cognitive/Brain:

◊   Decreased motivation and follow through
◊   Difficulty making decisions using logical reasoning
◊   Decreased alertness and concentration
◊   Decreased attention and working memory (both vital in learning and storing new information)
◊   Impaired memory (recalling stored information as well as storing new information since new stuff is only stored in the brain during sleep)
◊   Difficulty learning
◊   Slowed cognitive reaction time
◊   Decreased sex drive

Personality:

◊ You become a real jerk
◊ You stop doing things you used to enjoy
◊ You become a real jerk

Any relationship you have with others will be taxed to its limits when a new baby arrives, but especially with your partner if you have one. Everyone is tired, feeling incompetent, confused, frustrated and literally just holding it together by the sticky straps of a dirty diaper. So, when someone tells me they want to have a baby to "fix" a relationship I chuckle to myself and pray for the sake of the couple and potential new baby that they figure stuff out before/if the baby comes.

My partner and I are a strong couple. No, I'm not trying to brag or boast. Yes, many times I still ask myself, "What am I doing with this person?" when we don't see eye-to-eye on things. Regardless, I will share one huge secret with you as to why we have such a strong partnership. We respect each other. We love each other too, don't be silly, but we respect each other and see each other as our own individual persons with views that won't always agree. Nevertheless, when ya'll are sleep deprived, things can get ugly right quick.

Be patient with yourself and those helping you raise your baby. Be understanding that you won't always say the right thing or hear others' words the way they were intended. Know that you *will* survive, and your sacrifice now will be measured in many restful nights of sleep when they are older (usually around 13-20 months children tend find their night-time groove). You can do this!

Chapter 8

BEDTIME ROUTINE
You had Better Get on Board or Be Ready for a Rocky Ride

THE IMPORTANCE OF A night-time routine cannot be overstated. The importance of a night-time routine cannot be overstated. The importance of a night-time routine cannot be overstated. This is different from sleeping patterns. This routine is what you do with your child BEFORE they go to bed, and it alerts their little brains that it's time to wind down for the day.

From the first day our kids came home from the hospital they had a bedtime routine. No joke. When they were still breastfeeding the routine was bath, boob, and bed. Once they were weaned (Arthur self-weaned at 10 months and Ivy was encouraged to wean around 14 months for my sanity), the routine was bath, books (snack during books), then bed. I pored over many articles about sleep, I love sleep, and my best friend's doctorate dissertation was on circadian rhythms (sleep), so I know its importance and value (and yes, this is the BFF who threatened me within an inch of my life if I didn't stay awake all night for her birthday).

The bottom line for babies and young kids is this: babies and toddlers benefit from an early bedtime (in bed by 6/6:30 PM, *not* starting the routine at this time). Our routine would start at 5/5:30 some days. This also means they wake up sometime between 5 and 6:30 AM.

So, what are you? A morning person or a night owl? What is your child? Yes, genetics definitely play into this, but environment can also shape an individual who isn't strongly one or the other. Remember, self-knowledge matters because you have to learn and figure out your child's natural tendency, and then set a routine and sleep space times for them to get the recommended daily amount for their age. Your baby is a unique individual who you have to learn about and study in order to effectively parent and teach.

Having your baby in bed by 6:30 PM seems an impossible time frame! It may in fact be impossible for families with single parents or those with two working parents to keep this schedule. However, there are many families out there who *could* make this happen by shifting things. If you are one of those families, I doubly encourage you to shift shift shift.

My partner was not pleased with the early-to-bed routine as it meant she wasn't able to see the children in the evening after work due to her work hours. I hear this complaint from all my working parents and even the part-time working parents which say they don't feel they "see" their children enough.

I get it, I understand, yet I am just sharing what the research says and how it has impacted our family. A truth that arose from shifting the bedtimes earlier was that the time my partner ended up spending with the children in the morning was better in both *quality* and *quantity* than any time she would have gotten with the kids at the end of their day.

I remember when Arthur was in his first few months of life and my partner would race home from work to try and be home before 7:00 PM. I would have done my best to prepare a home cooked meal and we would sit and inhale it as fast as we could whilst Arthur fussed in a bouncer, tired and ready for bed, at our feet. Can't say I really enjoyed those evenings, nor did I digest my food well. But that's what we did until I read enough articles about early bedtimes, had observed and learned more about Arthur's cues and natural tendencies, and decided that it was what the kid needed.

I would have to say that when they were around 15-18 months old, and countless hours of sleep deprivation and sacrifice later, both my children started sleeping 10-12 hours through the night consistently. They would have the occasional night terror and need a quick cuddle or sometimes they were sick, but otherwise the children were in bed after books and either listened to children's stories or nursery rhythms via a CD, or to relaxing music without lyrics.

Never use TV or visual digital devices as a tool to get your child to sleep. All research suggests that this is counterproductive and actually stimulates the brain. This goes for you too mom/dad; take the TV out of the bedroom.

One thing I found invaluable was using a white noise machine in the room where the children sleep. The "shhhhh" sound from the machine masks other noises which might otherwise wake your sleeping babe. If you travel or your child sleeps in different locations the white noise is also a good mental "cue" for your baby to know it's sleep time.

Remember, the importance of a routine cannot be overstated. The repetition of activities (bath, brush teeth, books, and bed), is both comforting and calming to babies and young children. They know what to expect and the repetition in turn builds/strengthens those neural pathways by teaching our little ones that sleep is nothing to be afraid of but rather something to relax into and enjoy.

Chapter 9

BABY AND EVENING SLEEP

It Sucks For a Year at Least. Cope

YOUR LOVELY LITTLE BABY/TODDLER has been washed, powdered, diapered, dressed in pajamas and is ready for bed. They are, I think, at their cutest during this moment, *if* they are snoozy… but if they are overtired and wired they are not, I repeat *not* cute at this moment. Instead, they are little gremlins.

For the first year of their lives both my children preferred to sleep with, on, or near me, and as I have said and believe, as a parent you need to do your utmost to give your baby *anything* they want for the first 365 days. If this means co-sleeping to breastfeed at night so baby and mom sleep longer, great. If this means co-sleeping with toddler so the parents sleep "less" interrupted, great. I co-slept on several occasions when I was breastfeeding both children, but personally found it easier to sleep when my children were safely tucked into their own bed. Not only did I have more room to move around, I was also able to fall into a deeper sleep not worrying if I was going to roll over onto the baby.

Let's focus on those first 365 days again. During this first year of their life you are trying to lay a positive and healthy foundation for sleep. This isn't just about the physical but also the emotional part of teaching your infant that sleep is nothing to be afraid of and is actually an enjoyable place to be. You want them to know sleep is OK, you will be there when they wake up, you will take care of their needs when they cry out in the darkness, and you will be fast to respond so they do not have to fear sleep.

Some parents are lucky and have babies who sleep for long periods during the night. I wasn't one of those lucky parents. Obviously, infants will wake to be fed and as they get older they need fewer night feedings. They also wake up if they have gas, or something aches, or they just need a cuddle.

When mine woke to eat I would try to feed them in bed so I could sleep/rest longer, but those little stinkers preferred me to feed them in the recliner rocking chair. After many attempts to feed them in bed I gave up. What I learned was when I gave them what they wanted it meant the likelihood of them having a better/longer stretch of sleep increased dramatically.

Did this totally blow chunks for me? Oh, yes it did! Did this mean I slept like total crap for almost 3 years straight? You betya! Did people tell me all the time that what I was doing wasn't right (i.e. not letting my babies cry it out)? Damn straight they did! Did I listen to any of them? Not really. After the little ones were given what I *knew* they wanted, both of mine would usually sleep another 2-5 hour stretch before needing to feed again. To be honest though, after their initial 4-6 hour stretch the rest of the night was usually spent rocking and feeding during those first 365 days.

That being said, even if your child falls into a great pattern, it may change from time to time when they are mastering a new skill, and during times of regression (acting younger than they are). Remember, these are all a normal part of development. So, when things feel like they are sliding backwards just remember it's normal and will pass.

In general, evening sleep with a baby for the first 365 days is often a bumpy ride. I gave up a lot of sleep to make sure my children were given as many chances for sleep as possible. What I got in return were bags under my eyes, difficulty losing baby weight (research states it's harder to lose weight when sleep deprived and stressed), more grey hairs *and* two babies who learned by 15 months that night-time sleep is good, safe and when they wake they are able to turn their night light turtle toy on and go back to sleep by themselves. For me the sacrifice was worth it.

Chapter 10

WHO'S CRYING NOW?
My Opinion on the "Cry it Out" Method

MOST PARENTS OF A child under the age of 12 months are sleep-deprived. The extent to which you can survive/cope for a year without sleep depends on many variables that include, but aren't limited to: age, gender, genetics, natural sleep cycle, etc. Don't kid yourself. There are NO easy, long-term fixes you can do to make your baby sleep even though it seems many claim they have the "new-and-improved-get-that-cranky-baby-to-sleep-for-a-minimum-of-10-hours" solution for infants and sleep.

One of the most debated techniques to get babies to sleep is the "cry it out" method. Currently, there are many variations of this method, some less severe than the "leave-them-in-their-room-for-12-hours-straight" method. I did NOT use this method on my children, but I *did* think about it, and even *contemplated* doing it a few times when I was completely at my wits' end. Everyone's life is different with unique circumstances, and I am not here to judge anyone's choices. I'm here to share my knowledge.

What essentially happens when you sleep-train a baby is that the baby cognitively learns their cries will no longer be responded to and they simply shut down and stop asking (crying) for help from their caregiver. This small little human doesn't learn to self-soothe as previously thought, they simply learn that no one will answer their cries in the dark and so the behavior of crying stops/extinguishes.

Extinction is a behavioral technique used to stop a behavior (crying) when the behavior is not reinforced (leaving them alone in their crib). It should be noted that the amount of stress hormones (cortisol) released in an infant's system during a cry-it-out session can take up to 2-3 days to fully leave their bodies. And every time they "master" a new skill such as sitting, rolling, teething, or get sick, you will more than likely have to do a few "reminder sessions" and let them cry-it-out again.

Many physicians believe that babies are physically capable of sleeping through the night. If babies were a machine like a robot perhaps I could get on board, you know like the robot has enough battery power to last through the night. The problem is our babies aren't machines/robots. They are complex living, existing, breathing creatures that are more than just skin and bones, but soulful, spiritual and emotional beings.

I've read about a pediatrician in New York City who tells his patients that babies as young as 8 weeks old (that's 56 days people… 56 DAYS old), can be left alone for as long as 12 hours if necessary until they fall asleep. I'm not a medical doctor so I can't comment one way or another if it is physically possible. However, I can make a strong argument as a psychologist and mother that it is *not* the best way for you to build a trusting strong bond with your child, nor does it teach them to self-soothe. Plus, it feels completely unnatural.

As a psychologist my focus is not necessarily on whether or not a baby can physically survive for 12 hours without food. Lord knows my body can barely survive 2 hours before I see what helpless tidbit is gonna be eaten in my fridge. Emotionally speaking there is no way someone can argue with me that my 56 or 180 or 200-day-old baby is cognitively capable of understanding and developing healthy coping strategies to deal with the fact that when they cry out (in pain/fear/loneliness), I, their trusted guardian/mother/caregiver deserts them to fend for themselves.

Just typing that sentence sounded ridiculous to me. An individual's frontal lobes (think reason part of the brain), don't fully develop until 21 years old. Children don't even begin to understand metacognition (thinking about thinking), until roughly around 20-24 months. If your baby cries it out and then stops, they aren't developing coping skills. They are learning that no one will come when they cry.

At some point around 13-16 months old, when I knew my kids could cognitively understand the idea of "get your butt in bed it's time for sleep", I would let them fuss and cry for a little bit. Once, when Arthur was 14 months old, I let him "mad scream cry" for 15 minutes. After he calmed down, I went into his room to let him know I was here for him but that it was "bedtime". He was so angry that whenever I went into his room his cries doubled in sound. It was awful waiting for him to calm down again, so I could "check" on him. Remember, when you go in your child's room at the height of the scream you are reinforcing that level of crying so wait until they are quiet or calmer. I waited until he calmed down and then we chilled, had a cuddle and chat, and that was that.

Yes, even at 13-16 months I had to occasionally go into their room at night to help them get back to sleep, and by 22-24 months they slept in their beds no issues, and rarely have problems all night long. I told myself to put in the time early and crossed my fingers it would pay off when they got older. Both my kids love bedtime, they have no fear of the dark, they stay in their beds (they share a room), and they sleep 10-12 straight hours a night. They've been doing this since they were around 2 years old.

No, one, easy, quick fix exists for getting your baby to sleep through the night. Sometimes a parent is unable to constantly provide loving responses all night because they are a single parent who works in a factory around dangerous equipment (remember, if you are sleep-deprived your body responds the same way as if you've had a few drinks). I totally get that and can appreciate that. I simply ask that you examine your family's sleep needs and if possible, provide a constant support system for your baby during the first 365 days. It *will* pay off.

Chapter 11

NAPS
Yes, Please!

THE BIGGEST LIE OUT there is "nap when your baby/toddler naps." *ARE YOU KIDDING ME?* Whoever came up with this idea or even planted the seed for new parents that they can simply "catch up on sleep when baby sleeps" has obviously never had a newborn baby… or at least didn't raise mine. PLUS, the fact that as a full-time parent of a baby, a person's "alone" time decreases to about… well, nothing. So, when that baby is asleep and you are able to have a quiet moment (or at least a moment away from baby), I often found myself unable to sleep because I just wanted to be awake and not feel needed.

Our first child never wanted to nap unless he was in motion (pushed in a stroller or riding in a car), and my youngest was forced into her brother's nap routine due to convenience and the fact that she was more flexible in her sleep routine, unlike her brother. Let me explain.

Arthur, as you know, had colic and by the end of the day (when colic usually peaks), I would find myself out back bouncing in our hammock because he found relief in the movement and stopped crying for at least 5 minutes (which is priceless to a parent who has heard crying off and on all day). Also, I would be able to see the very second my partner walked into the backyard from work, which ranged between 6:30 and 7:30 PM.

Sometimes by 7:00 PM, having been alone with him since 8:00 AM, I was ready to literally throw in the diaper as a stay-at-home parent. I was mentally, emotionally and physically exhausted. Sometimes my partner didn't even get to walk in the house to drop off her bag and coat before I thrust Arthur into her arms.

When Arthur was 2 weeks old we found out my partner's mum was diagnosed with terminal cancer and was given 2 weeks to 2 months to live. She miraculously lived a full year and at the age of 2 months, Arthur, my wife and I were waiting in a line downtown Chicago at the Federal Building trying to get our newborn a passport because we were flying to the UK so my partner's mum could meet her first grandson.

I'm sure all the back and forth travel to the UK during Arthur's first year of life (4 round trips with each stay lasting between 14 to 22 days), combined with his colic and extreme sensitivity to sounds and lights, made it nearly impossible for me to know if he had never *found* his groove for his nap until he was around 12 months old because he wasn't given great "sleep space", or maybe he really did just *need* that much time to figure things out. Let's face it, that much international travel is tough on everyone.

Regardless of the cause, it didn't seem to matter what I did, that little stinker would wake at the slightest change in his environment from a flicker of light, a creak of the floorboards, or a dog barking across the street. For countless hours I sat in chairs, or on a bouncy exercise ball, or even pushing a stroller through the streets of Chicago during blizzard conditions just to try and get him to sleep. The only way I could get him to go to sleep outside of being in my arms or sucking on my boob was in the stroller or in his car seat as I drove around town.

About 2 miles from me in Chicago is a place called Rosehill Cemetery. This place has been around since the mid-1800s, it sits on 350 acres and boasts 23 miles of road. Before you think I'm macabre or odd when I say I spent a minimum of 2 hours a day driving in a cemetery for the first 10 months of my son's life, please note it was with purpose.

You know, or soon will, that when a child falls asleep in the car and you come to a stoplight, well that stoplight becomes a mortal enemy to you because if the car stops, the baby wakes. Rosehill has 5 stop signs in the entire cemetery, and lots of bumpy road that can be driven at 10 miles per hour by a sleep deprived new mother without fear of crashing the car or hitting a pedestrian. I even took people who came to see "the baby" for drives there when I needed him to sleep. As parents, we do whatever it takes.

As Arthur got older my challenge wasn't getting him to sleep in the car or stroller, it was getting him to slow his mind down long enough to fall asleep in his bed. He has always been very aware, curious and interested in his surroundings. It's a double-edged sword because it means his mind doesn't want to stop working to take a nap. Consequently, I had to become his external control "reminder" to turn off his thoughts. When he was old enough to comprehend what I was saying (around 1½-2 years old), I would say things like:

◊　　I know you are just learning your numbers/ABCs and it's fun to practice them, but I need you to shut off your mind and tell it "it's time to go to sleep".

◊　　Remember, our minds can only remember new information we've learned if we sleep. Because during sleep we sort and store that new information in our brains. (This is a true statement BTW. Sleep must happen for us to encode new information into our long-term memory.)

◊　　If you don't go to sleep, I will get very cross and you can potentially lose privileges. (Such as 20 minutes of TV, going to the park, playing a favorite game, etc.)

I honestly would say all of the above things to try to help him calm down and chill out. The words would be spoken in that "tone"; you know… the one that always meant business when your parents (authority figures), used it with you. Of course, when your child is pre-verbal they don't necessarily understand your words but they definitely understand your tone.

Once Ivy started napping in the same room as Arthur I decided it was easier for me to sit quietly in the chair in their room (sometimes for 45 minutes), to keep him in bed, quiet and away from the crib and Ivy. Like I mentioned, Ivy has no issues falling asleep but Arthur… oh, man… it was a battle of the wills for sure. It was a nightmare at the time and sitting in that chair trying to remain calm whilst your overtired young toddler presses buttons and pushes limits is almost more than some can take, and several times I lost the battle and my patience.

On those occasions (after the screaming and tears), I would first and foremost apologize for losing my temper. And then I would talk to Arthur about the importance of sleep and again explain why I would get so upset when he messes around. He was able to understand and make the connection (with my help), that on the afternoons he doesn't nap it's harder for him to control his impulses and he gets in more trouble. Again, I was highlighting the importance of sleep.

Since my children are close in age, I was able to get them on the same sleeping schedule. Ivy is flexible in whether or not she naps and always sleeps well at night, so I never stressed about making sure she got her sleep space. Arthur on the other hand, if he missed a nap the rest of the day was ruined. I'm not joking here, many parents I've spoken to agree that if their child misses a nap shit gets real, real quick.

Bottom line, babies and young toddlers *need* naps. They need you to help them figure out the best way to get them to sleep and teach them the importance of napping. Again, you want to be consistent in the times and locations they nap. They will fight the naps like all kids do because life is new and exciting as they are learning and growing so quickly. The first two things I always assess when my baby/toddler starts to act a bit naughtier than usual are 1. Are they hungry? and 2. Are they rested?

Chapter 12

BABIES GET MILK
Milk, It's What's for Dinner

WHEN I THINK ABOUT babies and food I think "KISS", or Keep It Simple, Stupid. If you're the biological mother of the baby, you have the option to breastfeed. If you're not able to breastfeed or don't want to, then high-quality formula will be the route you should take. After all your bills are paid and if you have some disposable income leftover, I would highly recommend finding and using the highest quality formula you can afford. Remember this little person has *sooooo* much growing to do and the fuel they receive should be rich in nutrients.

Please note that I am well aware of how costly formula is, especially the organic ones, so know that I'm not judging; I'm just sharing my two cents.

If you are the biological mother and you are adamant against breastfeeding, I'm totally fine with that choice... as it's your choice to make! My four cents on this is to share the following: breastmilk right after birth has a very special and important nutrient called colostrum that contains antibodies to protect your newborn against disease.

Your newborn could benefit greatly from their first few meals from your breast. If you are the biological mom and want to breastfeed, then wonderful... again it's your choice. It must be said that I do believe breastmilk is the best you can feed your baby. But it's not always possible for this to happen. Do your best; that's all anyone can do.

Chapter 13

BREASTFEEDING
My Experience, Enjoy

THE YEAR WAS 1999 and body piercings were just coming into style but were still somewhat taboo, at least in the Midwest. My best friend and I had pierced our noses in Philly (Philadelphia, PA) on a spring break trip the previous year and we were now ready to get another piercing.

Piercings are like tattoos I hear, once you get one you want more. She decided to get her eyebrow pierced and I decided to get my nipple pierced. I was just coming to terms with my bi-sexuality and preferred this piercing as I felt it gave me a "I'm a badass" edge *and* I could easily hide it away from my parents and Mormon friends who I felt might disapprove. (Quick side note: The Church of Jesus Christ of Latter-Day Saints formally ex-communicated me when I was 28 years old. I told my bishop I planned to marry the love of my life who happened to be female. However, that is a story for another day.)

I have always struggled to stay within the parameters of what people consider "normal" in American society… sometimes I just had to be different and I wanted to pierce my nipple.

I remember it like yesterday, lying on the table with my breast exposed, my nipple poking through a cold, metal clamp and right before the needle pierced my skin I shouted, "WAIT! Will I still be able to breastfeed if I pierce my nipple?" The girl paused, looked at me from behind glasses and a facemask and said, "I don't know, I think so," and then shoved the needle through my nipple. I won't go into graphic details, just know these 3 things: 1. I was this particular girl's first time doing a nipple piercing 2. She had an "issue" getting the jewelry through my newly pierced nipple and had to call the manager to do it for her, and 3. I didn't cry even though it felt like someone was literally ripping off my nipple.

Why did I need to share that story? Besides the fact that it's full of fun and interesting information about my past, I shared it because 18 years before I had children I knew I wanted to breastfeed my kids if I ended up having them. By the way, that girl ended up being right, you *can* breastfeed after you have a nipple piercing.

My whole life I knew I wanted to be a mother and I knew I was going to breastfeed. I never once thought, "What if my body doesn't produce milk?" or "What if my nipples get sore and raw and bleed and crack?" I just knew that no matter what, I was going to feed my babies from my boobs and that was that. I firmly believe that our minds are much more powerful than previously thought. Thinking positive thoughts can have a *huge* impact on how our bodies respond.

Let me share with you a sport related study that demonstrates the power of the mind. There was a study conducted by Dr. Blaslotto at the University of Chicago where a group of basketball players were divided into 3 groups and tested on how many free throws they could make. After the initial assessment, the first group practiced shooting free throws for an extra hour each day. The second group was asked to simply visualize making free throws, and the third group did nothing extra.

After a re-test the first group who physically practiced the shots improved by 24%. The second group, which merely visualized themselves making the shots improved by 23%! That's a *massive* improvement! All those guys had to do was imagine that they were swooshing each shot and it improved their game! The last group didn't improve.

Mind over matter. Listen, if you are contemplating breastfeeding but are unsure or nervous, try some mindfulness and relaxation, and consider giving it a try. I believe breastmilk is best for babies. I also strongly believe it's every woman's choice.

Now, back to my boobs. And if you are feeling uncomfortable about how many times I reference my breasts I think that you should take note of it and try to figure out why. If I was an alien and landed on Earth and didn't know the purpose/function of breasts and had to make a guess based on TV, magazines, movies, and advertisements, I would say something like "the purpose of breasts are purely for the sexual pleasure of man (or woman)." Breasts are seen as sexual objects. These "objects" aren't even connected to the whole (a woman's body) but viewed and sold as "parts".

I am so sick and tired of hearing from men *and* women that they are uncomfortable seeing a woman breastfeed their baby in public, and therefore *the mother and child* should remove themselves. That is just absurd to me. Breasts were designed to feed and nourish babies!

Arthur was 2 months old when we took our first international flight. During these first few months of breastfeeding my firstborn, I found it difficult to find a comfortable position for both him and me. It was even harder with a strange man sitting next to me at an airport with many people. I was sitting in one of those huge airport seats at O'Hare and struggling to get the "hooter hider" (there are many names for these things but essentially something that covers the boobs whilst you feed the baby, but it suffocates the baby and I found them difficult to use), to cover my boob but still allow myself to see Arthur.

I was completely "over" the boob cover and Arthur was over me trying to help him latch to my nipple without my being able to see him. So I just ripped off my hooter hider and didn't give a hoot about hiding my hooters anymore. My baby needed to eat and I needed to see him and I didn't care who was uncomfortable seeing me feed my son.

Quick side note for those who don't know, a newborn baby will not automatically be able to latch onto your nipple. Techniques were taught to me in the hospital on ways to get them to latch on, and even with the expert standing next to me offering advice, I still struggled at first to get my kids to latch.

Of course, with practice and commitment (whipping those hooters out anywhere anytime), both myself and the kids figured it out and they began to latch on their own within the first month without me squeezing milk out of my boob as I tried to get the nipple in the right position as I shoved it in their mouths. Pretty image, I know.

By the time we were in line getting Ivy's passport at the Post Office in Chicago when she was around a month old, I easily breastfed her while waiting. I did step to the side whilst my partner kept our space, but I was impressed with myself for being able to get an infant to latch and stay on whilst I held her in one arm, standing up in public. I know women have breastfed in much harsher conditions (war zones for example), than I will ever be able to imagine. Yet, in those early weeks/months of parenting you take the wins wherever you can find them.

Interestingly, every time I breastfed in public I was waiting, almost wanting/wishing for someone to try and publicly shame me. Maybe that's why nobody did, they could sense my "go ahead, make my day" attitude. It was as if my body language and face were saying "hell yes these are my tits and I'm gonna pop these huge size double H's out for my wee little baby to suckle so they can grow into big, strong, healthy people. So what you gonna do about it?"

I was never ashamed of breastfeeding and always would ask whoever was present if they minded, and 98% of the time they didn't. I did have a few occasions where the person said they would leave for a bit and come back and I was cool with that; at least they were honest. More often than not the people were interested in "how things were going." I found that many people have never been around a baby who was breastfed and they were mainly curious about the process and how it works. And I've always said to someone, "If you have the guts to ask the question I will answer it. I will be honest so be ready for the response."

Like I've said before, I felt like I researched *everything* associated with infants/babies, which of course included breastfeeding. By the time Ivy was coming off the boob and due to the fact that the children were 19 months apart, I had been breastfeeding for about 3 years straight. I did have a small 9-month break between when Arthur self-weaned and when Ivy picked up the habit 9 months later. What I found in my research and self-study was that everyone has different experiences with breastfeeding, and that doesn't surprise me.

What *did* surprise me was how many of the websites made me feel like there was only one way to breastfeed and it was *their* way, especially when it came to how soon to introduce a bottle, having a pacifier, etc. It became easy for me to see how women stopped breastfeeding; the stories my friends told me echoed my research. One can easily become overwhelmed with feelings of inadequacy and anxiety associated with stress about your ability to feed and nourish a baby.

I feel media and social pressures deter women from breastfeeding. Plus, in American society during the first half of the 20th century, formula advertising used subtle and not so subtle ways to sell the idea that formula is better for baby and mother; they did this by playing on insecurities and anxieties, and outright shaming in their ad campaigns. These formula companies also donated samples and pamphlets about the negative aspects of breastfeeding to new mothers in hospitals.

The idea that a woman's own breast milk wasn't good enough and that they didn't need to breastfeed anymore increased as more and more women picked formula over breast milk. In the 1900s nearly all women in the USA breastfed, but once formula advertisements and free samples were given to new mothers in hospitals there was a marked decrease in breastfeeding and an increase in giving formula.

More women were having babies in hospitals rather than at home which increased formula's "exposure" to new mothers who were seeking networks and people who "knew what to do" with a baby. I'm not going to go on any more about how companies and social pressures shifted the notion that breastmilk was inferior to formula, but I'm happy to say breastfeeding is currently on a significant rise in the States.

Whether or not you breastfeed, the world seems to have an opinion on how LONG one should do it. Like I said, the first few meals would be amazing for every little baby to have from a boob, and I agree with physicians that breastfeeding for 12 months is a good *minimum* number, but physicians say for your child to have the maximum benefit of breastmilk you should feed them from the boob until they are 2 to 3 years old.

Arthur was over the boob at 10 months and I weaned Ivy at 14 months because I couldn't stand having a tiny parasite attached to me one more day, so I did the minimum recommendation. Whilst I was very happy to be done breastfeeding at 14 months, I could have easily been persuaded to breastfeed longer if my partner felt passionately about it. But selfishly I could only be bothered to breastfeed for 14 months.

Even though I was going to be home all day and my little parasite had access to my breast 24/7, I wasn't sure if I needed a pump. Given that I would want a break from the babies *and* wanted them to only have breastmilk (as time goes on you'll notice some of your "musts" get mushy), I decided to pump. To be honest, Arthur was on my boob so much during the 10 months he breastfed that I didn't feel I had enough of a break in between feedings to pump.

When I did get a second to pump, I quickly became frustrated and felt like a failure because I could only produce 1, 2, or 4 ounces of milk. I also thought that if I wasn't pumping much, it must mean that my baby wasn't getting enough to eat. NOT TRUE! A baby suckling a nipple is totally different than a machine squeezing and suctioning milk from your body. I definitely have increased empathy for dairy cows. The amount that comes out from a machine is not indicative of how much your child receives. If they look healthy, are peeing/pooping normally, and are gaining weight, don't stress. Trust yourself.

Not only did I stop stressing about pumping and storage but I decided that if I wasn't around and he needed a feed, and I didn't have a pre-pumped bottle ready, then he could have formula. That "compromise" started out of necessity. Due to all the travel back and forth to the UK, my milk production cycle got outta sync.

Essentially, your boobs produce more or less milk throughout the day in accordance to both baby's needs and the time of day. I would have to say Arthur was fed 99% breastmilk and the occasional formula bottle. Ivy, well, that little stinker refused a bottle. When I would explain to people who wanted to feed her that she refused the bottle, people would pop up and say, "Well, I guess if she gets hungry enough, she will take a bottle." Yes, they are probably correct. But why? Why force her through that trauma when I am around and willing to sacrifice for the first 365 days. She got nothing but boob.

Both times the kids weaned my breasts were in serious pain. I thought since Arthur quit so quickly that that must have caused all the pressure and back up. So, when I weaned Ivy I thought dragging it out and giving her just a morning and evening feed would help with the pain. NOPE! Didn't help at all. The only thing that helped was cold, green cabbage leaves. Yup, tear off a nice leaf of it and put it in your bra. Truly a lifesaver.

During weaning besides the physical pain that you endure (and the hormone changes), there is an emotional feeling of loss as well. The closeness you have when feeding your child is very special. I tried hard to capture the feelings and experience of my "last feed" with Ivy knowing I would never have another baby suckle my breasts. Interestingly, I don't remember our last time, I just remember being aware that I would never again in my lifetime have this experience and to try and be grateful for the opportunity.

I made it sound like breastfeeding was a breeze. For the most part I found it easy, but every woman's experience is different. My nipples did get a little chaffed and red when the children were infants and just "breaking them in". Many creams exist for sore/cracked nipples and they helped a lot. Eventually your body will adjust to the constant sucking and your nipples stop cracking. I didn't have inflamed mammary glands, I never leaked in my bra, etc. Many women suffer with extreme pain when breastfeeding due to a myriad of reasons (infection, overproduction, etc.). I was one of the lucky ones whose experience was fairly straightforward and "textbook".

The last tidbit of information I will leave with you regarding breastfeeding is this. IT DIDN'T HELP ME LOSE WEIGHT! Granted, I wasn't counting calories and I wasn't restricting myself that much when it came to cravings. Yet, after researching much on this topic I found that I wasn't alone in my struggle to lose weight whilst breastfeeding.

The body is a smart machine, and I believe that for some women the body's metabolism slows down even more when they breastfeed. The body wants to conserve and hold onto every possible unit of energy since one person is essentially feeding two people. At least this is the story I told myself, so I could cope with my feeling like a failure because the baby weight wasn't melting off like I was told it would if I breastfed.

At times, I felt everyone else was able to do it easily and I was just a stupid fat loser that would never lose the baby weight within the recommended first year. I mean, in dealing with everything that comes with a new baby, the last thing I needed to stress about was losing weight.

I worked hard to let go of the stress about losing the 100 pounds I had gained and 4 years later, my tired body is still struggling to lose weight. I did manage to lose 70 of the 100 pounds I gained after my youngest was 2 years old because I was getting consistent sleep and was able to take exercise walks in the morning. I attempted to make myself feel better by saying that at least the kids' memories of snuggles with me will be all "squishy, soft and cozy."

Chapter 14

TRANSITION FROM MILK TO MEALS

Baby-led Weaning or Pureed Protein

MY PARTNER IS FROM the UK and I've learned over our 12-year relationship that just because you speak the same language doesn't mean you share the same culture. Much of Europe/the UK and other developed countries believe in a method of weaning, very cleverly called Baby-led Weaning.

In short, Baby-led Weaning (BLW) is skipping thin and runny purées and not feeding your baby with a spoon. Baby-led Weaning means offering your baby age appropriate foods that are soft-cooked and cut or mashed into small easily manageable pieces.

Side note: Arthur's first food was a banana, he loved it, he inhaled it, and we probably let him eat more than he should have for the first time but we had wanted my partner's mum to witness him eating for the first time and they both loved the experience. However, banana binds up your bowels, making it very hard to poo and is known for causing constipation. The saying in the lunchroom at the nursing and rehabilitation hospitals I worked at was "give 'em bananas, give 'em prunes".

Yup, poor baby Arthur (who was around 7 months old at the time and on his third UK visit since birth), was constipated. He was my colicky baby who had digestive issues anyway and he had eaten almost

¼ of a banana, which is a lot for their tiny tummies. My partner and I were racing around trying to find a pharmacy that was still open. It was a culture shock to come from America where there is at least one 24/7 pharmacy nearby to, "Oh, I don't know if anything will be open at 10:00 PM," with a screaming infant in the backseat of the car. Small, small culture shock.

Regardless of Arthur's and our first experience with Baby-led Weaning, I knew I wanted to move forward with this method. First of all, I try really hard to put myself and my mind into that of my child's. Would I want to eat some of the baby food you can buy at the store? The pureed meat mush? No, I wouldn't. So why would that be the first thing I introduce my child to when it comes to food? Food is something that brings pleasure and comfort, not only physically, but often emotionally and socially too.

I believe the first year of their life, a baby's primary source of nutrients/food is breastmilk/formula. Let the introduction of solid foods begin around 6-8 months (I'm reading more and more scientific papers stating parents are introducing solid/pureed foods too early which in turn is leading to an increase in food allergies and digestive issues).

Plus, what's the rush to feed them solids? Unless you have a physician telling you your child is underweight and his food intake needs supplementing with solid foods, don't stress how much or what they eat. Simply offer them a variety of foods in their purest forms which are soft enough or small enough to not choke on.

Back in the day when our ancestors were wearing animal skins, they weren't pureeing food for their babies. Though yes, they may have done what is called premastication: pre-chewing food for the purpose of physically breaking it down in order to feed another that is incapable of masticating the food by themselves. Essentially, bird-feeding your kid. Imagine eating a bite of your dinner, chewing it and then giving the food to your child to eat.

At the end of the day what I'm merely trying to say is that before blenders and mixers, our ancestors survived by doing either what's called "Baby-led Weaning" or premastication. So, if you wanna try it but are one of those people who tend to be nervous, curb your anxiety if you can and give it a try.

Know that your child's palette will change on a dime and each child is different. Ivy loves smoked salmon with lemon. Smoked salmon is very expensive; especially at the rate our daughter packs it away. So I budget the groceries to make sure we always have it in the house because it's so healthy.

Arthur used to like smoked salmon and then one day when he was around 13 months, he stopped eating it. Don't take it personally when your little one suddenly stops liking something, that's normal. Just try to roll with it and find something else your child will eat.

Don't make yourself crazy trying to come up with a new dish/food for every meal of every day. I know from experience… it will drive you mental and it's not worth it. The better, more manageable and sane way I've found is to always have nutrient dense foods (cheese, fruits, veggies, dairy/yogurt), that they love offered for every meal and have one or two new things over the course of the day to introduce to them.

Kids (and adults) like what we know. Familiarity is important and once your child likes something, keep offering it, maybe in new ways. Eggs for example can be fried, poached, scrambled, or hard-medium- and soft boiled! That's variety, no? Eggs are one of the best things a young child can eat. For about 6 months in a row my family ate eggs, bacon, toast and fruit for breakfast every day.

Then the kids got tired of it so we changed it up to cereals and cottage cheese. But I still give them eggs at least 4 times a week. They tend to fight it more now, but I usually win. My kids also have had pasta every day of their life since they were little.

Pasta in my book is a good bang for your buck! Lots of nutrients, cheap, and the shapes and textures are endless. In this day and age pasta can be made out of a variety of different beans, legumes, or other vegetables. You also have a variety of toppings such as cheese sauce, marinara, an Asian soy sauce, butter and parmesan... You get my drift.

Knowing that at least one meal a day you won't be fighting to get your child to eat will be one less thing to stress about. Add veggies to it if you want or keep it super simple. At each meal I offer our children their food over 2-3 courses. The first course is the carb/protein/veggie portion, followed by fresh fruit and sometimes yogurt.

So that's basically it for me on food. Keep it simple and as close to the natural state as possible. Breastmilk is best, but parents can't always offer that. Don't start solids until around 6-8 months. Finally, remember "food before one is fun". Don't pressure your baby to eat solids too soon and try to enjoy the process of introducing different foods to your child.

Chapter 15

IN THE MOOD FOR FOOD
A Few Things to Snack On

I REMEMBER IT LIKE it was yesterday; you know those few and precious moments in your life when someone/something happens to you and the way you view the world is forever changed? The waiting room in the mental health clinic on Chicago's westside was anything but posh. I was 3 years into my doctorate program completing one of my clinical practicums; I felt confident and competent not only with my theoretical knowledge of working with families but also my professional interactions working with clients from primarily poor, black, urban neighborhoods. I had a few minutes before my newest client and I began our intake session, so I peered through the receptionist's window into the waiting room to see if she had arrived.

She had, along with 5 children under the age of 7. The eldest child was "in charge" of the younger ones whilst my new client filled out the intake forms. The youngest in the group was around 12 months old; she was wearing a saggy/dirty diaper, her clothes were 2 sizes too big and she was being fed hot *Cheetos* and drinking orange soda from a baby bottle. Let's just say *many* judgmental thoughts raced through my mind about this young woman and her parenting competency before I even met her.

During the intake I learned that this 17-year-old girl was not only the primary caregiver for her 2 children, but her brother's 3 children as well as her ailing grandma (with whom they all lived). She was a survivor of sexual, emotional, and physical abuse and dropped out of school at the age of 15. (She was currently in the process of completing her GED.) I also learned that this young woman was a survivor, a fighter, and a champion for women's equality; she had dreams of becoming a lawyer one day.

The moment that changed my worldview came at the end of the session. When I asked this obviously bright and thoughtful 17-year-old why the youngest girl was eating hot *Cheetos* and drinking orange soda pop she sadly but confidently said to me, "I can afford one gallon of milk or 3 liters of pop and ain't nobody wanna feel hungry."

I was speechless, I was humbled, and I was changed. Even though I was aware of my initial judgments and told myself to acknowledge them, my strongest reaction which was hard to shake was thinking that this young woman was selfish, unconcerned about her child's health and maybe not very bright. Wow, did I take a blow to the brain, and it's never been the same since.

Talking about food can be a "hot topic" to many people because, I believe, at some time or another everyone has had issues associated with food and drink. Women seem to be the ones in society whose relationship with food is more widely spoken about; nevertheless, men are increasingly feeling the body image stress that women have always felt since… forever?

I am not a nutritionist; I've not taken formal classes that look at food and its scientific relationship to the body and health. (However, I did take a few classes in my formal education that looked at poor health and its impact on mental health and the brain.) What I have been is roughly 20-50 pounds overweight my entire life with a BMI that lies in the obese range (even though I'm built like a brick house and as strong as a workhorse).

I told myself I was big boned and most of the people in my family carry extra weight so I never really stressed too much about it. Then when I was 26, I decided to try Weight Watchers and learned SOOOO much about food and my relationship with it (both negative and positive). I lost 50 pounds and became a lifetime member.

That experience forever changed my relationship with food and began my passion for learning about nutrition, health, and cooking. Weight is fluid and I've learned that I can't place all my self-esteem in some number on a scale. My relationship with food is now one of appreciation, understanding and frustration. I say frustration because I've not enjoyed taking so much of my "life" to measure food, count calories and think about food. I've lost years to this topic.

I share my past struggles with food because it directly impacts my current life and the life of my children. If I feel healthy and happy and am able to find time to prepare homemade meals and walk or exercise, I feel better and am happier and therefore have more resources to care for my children. Also, I don't want my bad food habits inadvertently being taught to my children. Kids see what their parents eat, when they eat, and *if* they eat. Modeling good eating patterns is important when instilling good eating habits in our children.

I can honestly say, hand over heart, that I have never *driven* through a fast food restaurant with my kids in the car for two reasons. First, the food quality is not the highest from fast food restaurants, especially those with drive-thrus. Second, I don't want to listen to my child begging to go to every restaurant they pass; I live in the city of Chicago, people, we got drive-thrus on every block.

This doesn't mean that when I'm *alone* in the car I won't occasionally grab a snack at a drive-thru restaurant, because I do. This also doesn't mean that I stopped eating the occasional bag of guilty pleasures; I just don't do it in front of my kids.

Kids force us to change whether we want to or not. Why not choose to change for the better not only for you but for your child? Food is one of the most important things in your child's life and it will be for the rest of their life. Teach them healthy eating habits early and if needed, change how you eat for the better.

Chapter 16

KIDS ARE CAPABLE
Expect More, Compare Less

I HAVE HAD THE pleasure of working with children with disabilities for over 20+ years. Being around families of typically and non-typically developing children has taught me just how much *all* children are capable of doing. Often, I found parents of children with disabilities tend to push their children to reach their fullest capacity because they know life is going to be much more difficult for their child.

While working as a music therapist, one of my contracts was at a school that served children with severe and profound disabilities including but not limited to: autistic spectrum, spina bifida, cerebral palsy, and severe profound intellectual functioning. Some of the children had one disability such as spina bifida, but most of the children had multiple physical *and* cognitive impairments. The school employs 4 nurses, 2 physical therapists, 2 occupational therapists, 1 speech therapist, 1 social worker and each classroom has 3 to 4 teachers and aids. Many of the children have a 1:1 aid to assist them with things like eating, learning how to grasp a spoon, and keeping their faces dry from excessive and uncontrollable drooling.

These beautiful children were having a blast at school and loved their teachers and aids. What I learned over the course of working at the school multiple days a week for over a year was this: even a child with severe profound mental and physical disabilities is still just a kid. They try to see what mischief they can get away with, they try to manipulate adults around them to get what they want, and they need to be pushed to reach their maximum potential.

I watched each child grow, change and improve. These improvements were measured very differently from a typically developing child. A goal could be as simple as a child making eye contact during a song or holding onto a mallet and hitting a drum. Holding a mallet and hitting a drum increases fine motor strength and therefore the control that helps them grasp a spoon to feed themselves.

When my oldest was 15-months and still very much non-verbal, he and I were out back raking leaves. Most of the leaves were brown or yellow, but we had a few brilliant red leaves. I noticed he was closely examining a red leaf in his chubby little hands. I asked him if he could find me another red leaf. He immediately bent over, rustled through the pile and found another red leaf! I was floored and thought maybe it had to be an anomaly. So I asked him again to find another red leaf, and he did.

Your little baby has much more going on in their brains than we adults could ever really fathom. Something you can do as a parent to communicate with your child before they are verbal is to teach them sign language. I taught Arthur a few signs that I thought would help communication such as "more", "please", "thank you", and my all-time favorite, "chill out" (i.e. wait).

Did you also know that over 80% of all communication is nonverbal? That means eye rolls, slouchy stances, hands on hips, and biting lips all have meanings deeper than the words often used to communicate the meanings behind these gestures. A baby isn't gonna smack her lips or roll his eyes when you tell them to calm down. Their body language will tell you what they need; the tricky part is learning how to read it and that simply takes time and focus on your part. From the first day you bring your new baby home, try looking at them as if they were a small human rather than a baby.

Babies are often associated with dolls. Dolls don't have rights, dolls aren't expected to express themselves, and dolls don't have emotions and feelings and needs. Dolls are there for us to play with on *our* time and on *our* terms, not theirs. We own dolls. They have to obey and they never talk back. Can you see where I am going with this? Reframing how you view your baby helps how you interact with them and your overall expectations: tiny little human beings with individual needs and wants vs. a baby doll to dress up to show off.

Remember, every child develops at their own pace. Online websites can be wonderful resources, but they can also stress you out if you start comparing your child. Don't find yourself too bogged down with the exact week/day a typically developing child *should be* rolling over or start crawling. Obviously, if your baby is months behind on a benchmark then I would advise you seek out professional advice. Try to be as chill and Zen as you can be during the first 2 years. Don't over complicate things unnecessarily.

I know, I know, it sounds like I am talking out of both sides of my mouth but I'm not. What I am saying is as you watch your baby grow, remember they are little people and capable of doing more than you think, but don't stress if they don't hit benchmarks set-up as guidelines on websites.

Your young toddler is capable of impulse control, waiting, empathy and entertaining themselves. When mine were a little over a year old they started doing chores like assisting with emptying the dishwasher and feeding the dogs.

I don't play when it comes to everyone chipping in and pulling their own weight on the family ship. It's important to instill a sense of teamwork, belonging, ownership and accomplishment from a young age. Your children will flourish in an environment of support and learning. Yes, a 10-minute job can quickly become a 30-minute job when little hands are helping. Just remember those extra 20 minutes are an investment in your future. You are instilling in your child's motherboard (brain's neural pathways), not only fine and gross motor skills but also a sense of togetherness and the satisfaction one gets when standing back and looking at a job well done.

Chapter 17

IT'S NOT WHAT YOU SAID, BUT HOW YOU SAID IT
How to Use Your Words and Tone of Voice to
Lay the Foundation for Executive Functions

REMEMBER WHEN YOUR MOM (or an authority figure), would force you to apologize to that "little brat" who took your favorite toy and sneered at you the minute your mom turned her back? It took lots of inner strength to utter the words "I'm sorry". We did it because we didn't want to get punished, but we sure didn't mean it! I don't know how it was for you, but in my house after I had finally uttered those two magical words and started to walk away my mom would say, "Do it again, Bethany... change your tone and mean it." It always started an argument between us because I would argue, "I said what you wanted," and my mom would say, "Yes, but your tone said you didn't mean it," to which I would respond, "WELL OF COURSE I DON'T MEAN IT! I HATE THAT KID!"

Think of your tone of voice more like an attitude. The words in a sentence can have other meanings besides the original meaning of those words depending on the sound of your voice. I wasn't really apologizing to that brat, and anyone who heard me say "I'm sorry" knew I wasn't truly sorry.

When it comes to babies/children and communicating with them, remember it's all about your tone. In other words your ability to convey what you want simply by changing the sound of your voice.

I remember when the kids were 12 and 21 months old and I was in the other part of the house (translation: I was taking a poo in the loo), when I heard an argument breakout between the kids. It was around this time in their relationship that Arthur enjoyed shoving Ivy, who was still mastering how to walk. It doesn't matter how much you babyproof your home; if shoving begins on unsteady feet, someone is gonna get hurt. I was seriously, like mid-poo, and could not jump off the toilet to intervene. Instead I shouted with my deepest, loudest and most authoritative voice three words they both have heard before: "HEY. STOP. NOW." Guess what, it worked. They stopped immediately. It wasn't magic; it was my tone, pitch and volume. More specifically, the words initiated what's called the "acoustic startle reflex" in the children.

The area of the brain that gets triggered when someone shouts using short, loud, sharp tones is called the limbic system. The limbic system is composed of various structures in the brain that deal with emotions, such as sadness, anger, happiness and fear, as well as memories and arousal states (think stimulation).

Think about a time when you were out in public minding your own business and suddenly you hear someone shout, "HEY!" and you immediately stop whatever you are doing and turn to see who it was and if they were talking to you. In that split moment, the other person was able to totally derail you mentally by initiating the acoustic startle reflex with a short verbal "punch" to your brain in the form of the word "hey". We turn around and look automatically because it is prewired in our brains to do so for survival reasons.

If someone is crossing the street and not paying attention to traffic, they may not see a car turning in front of them. But if someone shouted "Hey!" loudly, this individual is more than likely going to stop looking at their phone and look up to assess for danger.

Your tone and volume can cause a momentary "pause" in someone's brain and open up mental space to receive new information. Was that person who shouted "HEY!" actually talking to you? Did they break your concentration? Did your heart start pounding a little bit after you realized you weren't in danger (because it can also start your brain's survival responses of fight/flight/freeze)? Maybe you even felt a little silly for turning around? At the end of the day, you've survived until now because your body is responding in the way it is programmed to respond.

Now, let's talk about how to use the body's natural response to our advantage as parents. Pick a word, other than "no" that is short and easy for you to say loudly and sharply. The reason I don't want you to use the word "no" is because sometimes you simply want to grab your child's attention and not necessarily say "no" to the activity they are doing. Personal favorites of mine are the classic words "hey" and "yo". Let's practice with the word "hey". I want you to say it the following three ways.

Long and loud and let the sound trail off at the end: HEEEEEEEEEEEEEY.

Loud but not quite as long again letting the sound die down at the end.
HEEEEEeeeeY.

Now do it the loudest you've shouted thus far and make it short, stopping the sound abruptly.
HEY!

I'm not kidding when I say ask your partner or a friend to listen to you and let you know when they think you've got it down. I say this because a close friend and fellow psychologist, whose children are similar in age to mine, was struggling to get her very active son's attention when he was misbehaving or about to do something dangerous.

During a play date we were discussing this very topic and her son was, wait for it, misbehaving and not listening at all to his mom as he was climbing near a fireplace with sharp edges. We used the moment to "practice" the idea of mine and she tried saying "hey" to stop him and grab his attention. But after several attempts, she was unsuccessful. She looked at me and shrugged her shoulders and I said, "Do it again but louder." She did. "Even louder," I told her. She did. "LOUDER, MATE, LOUDER! FOR THE LOVE OF GOD, SHOUT!" Okay, I didn't quite say the last bit word for word, but she is soft-spoken by nature, and it did take her several attempts until she finally spoke loud enough and with enough authority to jolt his limbic system, and then he stopped. Be prepared that the jolt will initially cause your baby/young toddlers to cry and that's a normal response. The world is still very new and until they start to learn and understand the world around them, new things which startle them often can trigger the fight/flight/freeze response; hence the crying.

Afterward, she said to me that she had no clue how loud she needed to be. In her mind she was shouting at her 19-month-old son, but what I heard as an observer was what I would label a "raised voice with mild concern" in her tone. She definitely was not shouting, and if I was being naughty and she tried to redirect my behavior with that tone of voice I would have just kept on being naughty, and I told her so. We laughed and cried at just how hard and awful being a parent is sometimes.

When you mean business with your child, mean business and don't mess around. Kids thrive in environments where boundaries are clear and consistent. That's why I want you to practice this with your partner or friend until you find the right tone and volume. Your practice partner will feel it when you hit their limbic system even if they are prepared for the noise. That's when you know you've got it down!

What you don't want to do, now that you understand how to grab your child's attention, is to over use it. Each time you derail your child's attention by hitting the limbic system it can set off the fight/flight/freeze response in their brain that in turn releases the stress hormone cortisol which isn't great for a baby's system in high doses.

When your child is a baby/toddler knowing how to do this effectively may save your baby from a fall, a broken bone, or even save their life (think walking in front of a moving car). Just don't overdo it to the point that your child becomes full of stress hormones and fearful of exploring the world around them.

This brings me to the next step in the process. You might notice with yourself and/or your children, that right after the startled effect of hearing "hey!" wears off, there is a brief pause while the brain assesses if the danger is a real threat or not. This pause in babies is short and sometimes hard to catch before they go straight to tears. Like I said, if you are using it to stop your child from touching a hot stovetop then their natural response to cry after you yelled, "HEY, NO!" is totally fine and much easier to deal with than a burnt hand.

As they get older you will begin to notice the "pause" time increases slightly. This is usually when their desire for something is so strong that the jolt to their limbic system doesn't completely derail them and you have a few brief moments, literally seconds, to try to redirect and refocus their behavior, this in turn builds the neural pathways needed down the road for executive functions like self-control, motivation and judgement.

During these precious moments it's important that your energy and tone of voice is calm and reassuring as you redirect their attention. Yelling, or a rough tone of voice, will definitely send them over the edge to tears. So, after you shout your attention-grabbing word, immediately soften your tone and level of volume. Using soothing sounds and soft touches also helps keep your little one focused on how they should change their behavior to get what they want.

Simply speaking, the back of your brain houses the cerebellum which is responsible for the fight, flight, or freeze response system in your body. The middle part of our brain houses the emotions (the limbic system). The front part of your brain houses the frontal lobes which give us our executive functions such as judgment, logic and reasoning.

When we are emotionally triggered or fearful, the front of the brain fights for control but the back of the brain usually wins. Imagine the last fight you had with someone, when you were really worked up. Your choices in those moments when you were driven by emotions may not have been the wisest ones. When your baby or young toddler is in the back of his brain with emotions (survival mode) there is nothing you can do but wait it out. Trying to talk to them during this time will accomplish nothing. They can't process anything you're saying, even if it's, "Stop crying and I will give you chocolate." It's impossible.

As a parent I think one of your primary jobs when raising a human is to help them build strong neural pathways for self-control. Think about the neural structure in the brain as a road system. There are highways, side roads, off ramps, and dead ends. The highways are paths that have been traveled the most thereby increasing their size and strength.

Think of one huge super highway running from the front (executive functions/frontal lobes), to the middle (limbic system/emotional center), to the back of the brain (primitive brain with only 3 response options: fight, flight, and freeze, your basic survival methods).

At times of serious distress, we (humans) need to be able to respond without using our frontal lobes to properly process a situation. Like if a cougar suddenly pops out of the woods near you, your body will more than likely respond without thinking anything at all. This super highway is needed for survival purposes but sadly gets used all too often as a way to cope with stressful or difficult situations.

It is during these early stages in infancy/young toddlerhood that you begin building and developing the foundation for how your baby will cope with stress for the rest of their lives. This is why you must teach them ways to cope and manage their fears, emotions and first experiences in the world in a positive and loving way. For little babies, to build their "off ramps" from the super highway, respond to them when they cry out for you. Every cry is a request for your attention as they are asking you to help them with something. It could be patting their back so they can burp, or holding them and kissing them when they get startled. By responding (even if you can't always stop the tears immediately), you are strengthening not only your bond with your child, but also the foundation from which their executive functions will further develop (judgement, reasoning, self-control, focus).

As your baby starts to get older and more cognitively aware of cause and effect, they can begin to develop coping skills (off ramps, to side roads and smaller highways), to prevent them from racing to the back of the brain and remain in control and/or neutral. One of the best techniques (research also touts the benefits) for calming down (no matter the age), is taking slow, deep, mindful breaths, and yes, counting to 10.

How do you teach mindful breathing techniques to someone non-verbal or just developing language? Tell your wee one to "smell the flower" (deep inhale through their nose) and then blow out the candle (slow exhale through the mouth), when they are calm enough to listen. Just like anything, the more you practice the better you become. This practice time needs to happen when your child is feeling happy and able to listen. You can simply say, "We are going to practice our calm/flower breathing now."

The trick to using this technique is being able to notice when your child is about to lose it and intervene *before* then. I'm not talking literally right before they throw something, but those few minutes beforehand when you notice they are beginning to struggle coping with frustrations, are not following directions, etc. It's in this moment when you can use flower breathing to keep them centered and in cognitive control.

Let's say that you had gone into the other room for a minute and come back to your 19 month old unrolling the toilet paper. No, this isn't the end of the world, but you also know your child is well aware that she is not supposed to do this. You do your quick "HEY!" to get their attention, then in the "pause" you softly and calmly say, "Listen, darling, you know you aren't supposed to do this and it makes me upset." They will most definitely be struggling to not cry at this point, then say, "Let's practice flower breathing and try to calm down whilst we pick up this mess." Then you calmly start to cleanup and hopefully your little one helps, too.

Let me give you another example of how to use "the pause" with a toddler. Arthur is my logical level-headed little guy. I rarely allow the children TV, but I do allow audio books. Whilst I love hearing children's stories, I don't want to hear them for hours on end; therefore, I've set aside a specific time of day when they listen to stories.

He has always been open to reason and has been successfully negotiating "one more time" quite well since he was 2 ½. That's because I reward him (reinforce the highway), when he is able to "keep it together" and listen, sometimes he does it on his own and sometimes he needs a reminder.

During an audio story time I had given the "this is the last one" heads up to try and minimize any potential upset. After the story ended Arthur started to cry. I said, "Hey!" loudly, which stopped the crying immediately and during that brief pause I quickly, softly and calmly followed it up by saying, "Arthur my love, if you would like one more story just say, 'one more please'. Don't cry to try and get what you want." At this point he hadn't completely lost control and I could see the cogs in his brain turning, so I again said, "If you can keep it together and say 'please' I will give you one more story." He took a deep breath, wiped his tears, and said, "One more, please." He got a *huge* hug, kiss and another story.

My goal as a parent isn't to make my children "toe the line". Yes, sometimes the "last time" will be just that. Regardless, my goal is to raise productive adults who are capable of self-regulation, self-awareness and self-control. It's about teaching them lifelong skills that empower them to make their own choices and to take responsibility for their actions. Of course, I'm not saying a 2-year-old is in complete control over themselves, but what I *am* saying is that we as parents have to teach this. We are naturally given thousands of chances during the day to try to teach self-control to our babes. And, no, not every single one of them will be teachable moments, nor will you have the mental capacity to make them teachable. Some days, it is seriously just about making sure no one gets hurt or dies.

If you yourself aren't good at self-control and keeping calm when you are triggered, then start practicing. You will find your relationships with others will improve. You will also develop more empathy toward your child as you teach them self-regulation/self-control which in turn builds a strong foundation for executive functions.

Chapter 18

STRICT WITHIN AN INCH AND FREE AS A BEE
How Clear Boundaries Create Independent and Creative Kids

I THINK BASEBALL HAD it right when they created the 3 strikes and you're out rule. That's the same rule I have in my house, even with babies/young toddlers. The two reasons I have a three-strike rule is 1. The first time you ask someone to do something there is a chance they didn't hear; even twice someone could have misheard. But three times? Na, you heard and you are actively ignoring my request. Not cool. Not OK. 2. I don't have the patience or the extra hours in a day to repeat myself multiple times.

Sometimes by the time I've had to ask twice I'm ready to snap. Yes, even when they are little and learning, you lose your patience. Nevertheless, during these first few hundred days of life it is important for you to set up clear consistent boundaries for your little one. Remember, kids are capable.

What can easily happen is that parents, wanting to be kind and loving, start out being lenient with rules and provide loose boundaries for their children, becoming stricter as the child ages. Logically, it makes sense, right? Be nice and fluffy with rules when they are little and helpless but be strict and firm when they are belligerent teenagers.

An example of boundary/rule setting with a baby/toddler could be not throwing toys. It's simple, when they throw a toy they get that toy taken away until they say (or sign) they are sorry and/or they may lose access to the toy for a day or two depending on age and what was thrown. Unfortunately, most parents I've spoken with feel they are being "mean" by setting limits with their young children.

In the semester breaks during my many years of college and graduate school, I used to substitute teach. One of the classes I was requested to teach repeatedly was a remedial high school math course. Let's just say in the early 2000s having a nose ring definitely gave me an edge.

Not only did the students respect me, but the staff was thrilled to have a substitute who could "manage" the remedial math class which is often filled with students who didn't want to be there and often suffer from a learning disability that went undiagnosed for some reason or the other.

I didn't do anything special. I merely came in and said something like, "Listen, we all know I'm not your regular teacher and I remember what it was like to have a substitute. We can have an awesome time in class or it can be complete and utter hell. It all depends on you as a group. If you aren't assholes, I won't be one either."

No, I don't make it a habit to cuss in front of high school kids. But I also don't make it a habit to underperform at a job. The nose ring and two cuss words had the kids thinking I was pretty fly. I came into the class with no slack on the leash. Over time, as I came to know the class and kids, I was able to let out the leash a little bit.

I've worked with many parents who tether their kids to a long leash and leave them flailing in the wind to try and figure out life. They don't do this intentionally (well at least the ones who aren't psychopaths), and they have good intentions at heart.

Many have said to me that they came from strict backgrounds and don't want to be that way with their children. Others had parents who didn't really know what to do, so they just left their kids alone for the most part. Of course, in this day and age the simple fact is that a person can grow up without being exposed to good parenting role models.

One time a client was in my office with her 8-year-old son who suffered from emotional and behavioral problems. She was at her wits' end and didn't know what to do. During the intake I asked her to describe what happens with her son during a meltdown. She shared that he "destroys my house." Often, household items are broken, including his toys. I asked her what happened to the toys that get ruined during these temper tantrums. She said, "I just replace them."

Nope, nada, NO! When your child, old or small, breaks a toy out of anger you don't replace it. After the meltdown subsides and everyone is in a place where they can process what just went down (sometimes my kids chill out before I am able to chill and recompose myself), it's important to say in that moment something like this:

I know you got upset and had a meltdown. I am glad you are now calm and we can talk about what happened. You should know I love you very much but I don't like what you did and I won't be replacing the toy you broke.

When you set a limit/boundary with your child the reinforcement and commitment to follow through as a parent must be strict within an inch of the rule. Much the same as bedtime is quiet time, and quiet means quiet.

When it's "free play" allow complete freedom in the least restrictive environment. It's vitally important that babies/young toddlers be given a minimum of one hour a day (spaced out throughout the day, think in 5-15 minute increments), in a setting that provides stimulation but which is also safe and doesn't require you to participate.

An example could be a playpen that is moved from one room to another or even outside weather permitting. This provides an opportunity for your child to be exposed to nature but in a safe way. As they grow into toddlers they will need more stimulation, so you could take them to a park.

Teaching and learning to respect limits are important to instill in your child(ren) and we parents have many opportunities to teach this throughout the day. When you set a limit it's important to stick to it and reinforce the rule. Keep in mind the rules need to be simple with babies and young children. We have essentially one house rule/mantra that covers almost everything:

Manners and kindness opens doors.

I came up with this when Arthur was about a year old. I thought long and hard about what was really the most important thing I wanted him to know and have embedded in his brain from early childhood, and it was this.

Life should be about becoming your truest self and about respecting the rights of others and Mother Nature. I'm teaching my young children that by being kind to others and using manners, many doors will be opened for them.

Personally, I can't tell you how many times my ability to say please and thank you or sending a thank you note to someone made all the difference in my relationships with others. Let's be honest though, no one likes being around someone who is a jerk. You know, those people who always tell one too many stories or jokes, or who never pay you back because, "Dude, it was only 3 dollars, relax." Being nice to people is important in this day and age, maybe even more than ever.

Aside from being nice and treating others with respect it's important that your little one understands the house rules. Keep the rules short and simple. Make sure the rules and consequences are consistent and clear. You will repeat yourself many times. You will repeat yourself many times. You will repeat yourself many times. That's how they learn, through repetition and being presented the same thing over and over again, but in slightly different ways. I am *still* telling my children to stop picking up stuff from the ground and putting it in their mouth.

Pick your battles, and even when your kid only takes one baby step toward a goal, be excited about it! I'm talkin' excited like confetti and balloons just dropped from the ceiling and your favorite dance jam just turned on excited! It will pay off instantly when your child smiles at you as you break into your "happy dance". When it's time to play, play. When it's time to set limits, set them and enforce them in kind and loving ways.

Chapter 19

TOO MUCH TOO SOON WILL BE YOUR DOOM

Less is More When it Comes to Toys and Activities

BEING A PARENT SOMETIMES feels like being the entertainment director on a cruise ship. However, being a parent when your kid(s) are babies brings it to a whole new level of "and *now* what do we do?"

Finding things to do with my young baby(ies) became a serious mental struggle for me. I woke every morning dreading the moment my partner left for work because it meant I was in charge of filling the rest of the day with things to do with my blobby baby/toddler.

One tried and true method many parents use to "fill the day" is by offering their infants/babies/toddlers screen time with TV or any touchscreen device. The American Academy of Pediatrics policy guideline discourages screen time for kids fewer than 2 years of age. However, it does make a distinction between *active* and *passive* screen time viewing.

Passive screen time is plopping your little one in front of something and leaving them there as you wander off to another part of the house to do something else and leaving the TV-iPad as the babysitter.

Active screen time is when you call your parent(s) and let your child Facetime/Skype with them during meals (because to invite them over either isn't practical due to distance or isn't practical due to the emotional disruption it will cause you to have them over). Even if you struggle being around your parents, it is always good to try and allow them to be grandparents to your kids if possible.

Arthur was probably 13 months old when I allowed him to watch ½ hour of TV occasionally. I was pregnant, tired and to be honest I thought he could benefit from it. I knew I had to be picky about what he watched and was looking for shows that had minimal stimulation. Shows where the cartoon characters don't even speak and instead just use non-verbal sounds and gestures. These shows can get a little boring for the parent.

Nevertheless, watch the shows through your child's eyes and you will immediately start to notice shows that you feel are "too much" for your little one to cognitively process. Remember, simple is what you're going for... if your child has never seen TV then a slow moving Claymation show is gonna knock their socks off. Don't start them out with some high definition surround sound experience cause you ain't gonna have enough Benjamins in your bank to keep meeting your child's expectations for excitement/entertainment.

You also want to search for shows that hold the same screen shot for a minimum of around 3 seconds. You will be amazed as you watch TV how quickly screenshots change in an effort to keep your attention. Babies and young toddlers can't process that much information flying at them all at once and quickly become overwhelmed and overstimulated.

Plus, it's not good for their brain development. Imagine the opening to any *Star Wars* movie where you're flying through space and it's utter darkness with white burning stars whizzing past your head. That's how a little one might experience a show with too much stimulation. Their brain just shuts down and can't deal, which usually results in tears.

Limited TV/screen time also means they have more "free" time to be outdoors. Some people argue that a touchpad device increases fine motor skills and hand-eye coordination. To that I will say yes, some studies have proven that a child with underdeveloped fine motor skills can increase their control by playing video games. But those studies were on children who were much older; I'm talking about kids under 2 here. Your babe needs to increase their fine motor skills digging in dirt, or playing with found objects (Tupperware, wooden cooking spoon, etc.), around the house not on a video game controller.

Bottom line: limit screen time as much as possible, *but* when you do allow them to watch TV or use a touchpad device, be thoughtful about it and consider why you are doing it (if this is a reward, did they earn the time? Or is this a break for yourself so you can have a bite of lunch alone out back for a full 5 minutes of uninterrupted bliss? Ain't no shame in that game, just be honest with yourself). Being aware of why you are using the TV will also help you plan for times when you actually need it.

For instance, this one time when the kids were 2 and 3 years old and my babysitter canceled last minute, and I had to take both kids to the dentist with me! I grabbed a laptop and two earphones and plopped their little buns on the floor at the foot of the dentist chair. They quietly sat and watched a movie for the 45 minutes it took to clean my teeth.

Limit screen time as much as you possibly can for as long as you possibly can. Soon enough they will be 5 years old and working on computers in school. If you do use screen time, be cognitively aware of why you are using it. Also, don't just leave your child in front of the TV, interact with them and listen to the stories that they are watching.

Often, I will find myself saying things like, "Do you remember on that show when the little bee was brave and got her shot at the doctors? Well, it's your turn to be brave and get your shot." Or they will be watching the TV whilst I am doing something else, like writing this book, and I will say something like, "Oooh, look at that big bug. After TV time let's go out and look for bugs."

Last thing about screen devices is this: NEVER ALLOW A TV OR SCREEN DEVICE IN YOUR CHILD'S BEDROOM! Research shows having a TV on in the bedroom actually stimulates brain waves and makes it harder to fall asleep. (That goes for you too, parents! Get the TV out of the bedroom.)

Most of the other primary parents I know (both personally and professionally), said one of the most difficult things about having a baby is filling the minutes and hours of a day. Let me tell you, those minutes and hours can, at times, seem unconquerable.

From the time you wake until the bedtime routine starts, it is usually the primary parent's job to fill the long long hours of being home with an infant or finding someone else to care for your child part of the day.

If your home has 2 working parents, then other people fill part of the day (i.e. grandparents, daycare, nanny etc.). For those who stay home full-time like I did, be prepared. Seriously, I was mentally living day to day and focusing on the minutes/hours so that I could cope.

I would wake and give myself a pep talk saying stuff like, "You can do this, you can make it through the day. You just have 12 hours to kill. You got it. One minute at a time." I kept hearing other people tell me the minutes feel like years, but the years will feel like minutes so enjoy them as much as you can. I really tried to take that to heart and at my lowest points would tell myself "…Girl, you got this. Ivy is not going to want to sleep on you the rest of her life, so just hang in there for another hour right now. Breathe, breathe."

What I ended up doing was shifting my perspective about time. I am the type of person who has a list of things I need to get done every day and I want to check things off my list as quickly and efficiently as possible so I can feel good about myself and feel like I "did something" productive during the day. Consequently, a HUGE shift in my perception of time was required.

For example, I live in a home which has multiple levels. One afternoon when Arthur was around 12 months old and I was 2 months pregnant with Ivy, I was tired and didn't feel like carrying him up the stairs *again*. Since we didn't have anything pressing to do, I let Arthur struggle and learn how to master the stairs. It took us around 15-20 minutes to climb one flight of stairs. But I wasn't lifting him, he was exploring and touching and feeling, I was killing time, and Arthur was learning valuable skills, getting exercise, and was happy.

Another example: I live in Chicago and believe in fresh air regardless of the weather and require the kids to be outside at least twice a day. When Arthur was just learning to walk, we would take one to two hours to simply walk around 1-2 blocks. He noticed everything from broken glass in the dirt, to flowers and dog poo. He seemed to have a keen eye for that, gross.

No, this was *not* the most riveting way I could be spending my afternoon, and many of my friends would load their days up with group music, swimming lessons or 'mommy and me' classes of any kind.

I asked one of my friends who worked part-time and had two children close in age to mine why she felt the need to have so many scheduled activities with her young babes. She said that it was because *she* needed to be around other mothers and those classes were for her sanity, not her sons'.

If you need to be around other people because it's too difficult for you to be home alone with your baby, I completely understand that need and the importance of meeting it. However, if you are scheduling more than 2 activities a week to do with your young one because you think *they* need it, stop. They don't need it.

When your babies are little and even when they start becoming toddlers, they engage in what's called parallel play. Meaning, they may sit next to another child but they don't interact and play together. What they *do* end up sharing are germs and bad habits.

Every single time I went to a "babies and me" class with all the other snotty-nosed babies, my little one(s) usually got sick and I ended up losing sleep for weeks due to one 45-minute activity. Nope, not for me so I stopped going. The lack of adult interaction did NOT override my hatred of dealing with sick babies. Consequently, I stopped going to activities that had more than 4-6 toddlers in them because I just didn't feel the benefit of my kids sitting next to another kid was worth the colds they inevitably caught.

The first 2 years of coping with your new life as a parent may feel like an eternity when you are living it. Try to present activities and exposure to the outside world at a slow and leisurely pace. Learn to slow down and find joy in watching your little one discover things by themselves. I found I didn't have to fill the days with activities but rather I had to fill the days with opportunities to explore in a safe and supervised area.

That made it more manageable for me mentally, to think about exposing them to opportunities to learn (finger paint with yogurt in a tray, pour beans and rice into two bowls and let them feel and explore them, etc.), rather than activities I had to lead and be in charge of.

Keep things simple as long as you can. It's hard, I can attest to that. But I can also attest to the fact that keeping it simple pays off tenfold in the long run. I'm not always looking for the next "best thing" to meet their high expectations of instant gratification and/or stimulation.

Pots, pans, wooden spoons, plastic bowls, lids and measuring cups. That's all you really need for the first 2 years of life. Honestly, I never bought a gift for our kids until they were around 3 years old. Others have purchased gifts for our children, sometimes they ask what I think the kids will like, but for the most part they play with what they have and we have plenty.

When they were infants, I was given a couple of play mats. The mats were helpful and both my babies laid on them for a few minutes at a time, gradually building up the length of time they could entertain themselves. It was also during play mat time that I took their diapers off. Yes, sometimes they peed on the mats (use puppy liners) but think about how hot their bums must get in a diaper all day, and how freeing it must feel and what a great experience it must be for them to be naked for a few minutes a day to explore.

Not only is it important to keep things simple from a toy perspective, but also from how much work you have to do. This is when things can get tricky, so listen carefully.

Your baby will benefit from as much time as they can tolerate on their own during a day. To clarify, choose times during the day when your baby is at their "best". This means all their needs have been met (food, sleep, poo), and they are simply looking for some stimulation for a few minutes.

During this time, you put them down someplace safe with a few age appropriate toys to explore. Between the age of 4-7 months babies begin to develop a sense of what has been termed by psychologists as "object permanence". This is when babies begin to realize that people and things still exist even when they're out of sight.

It was a day I will always remember, the day I was able to put my 5-month-old son on the floor and prepare dinner. I was able to walk in and out of his field of vision without him needing me. I love cooking; it's my mindfulness exercise of the day. When I wasn't able to cook due to a baby needing attention and no one else to provide it, I was honestly miserable.

As I slowly began to build Arthur's tolerance for entertaining himself, I was also getting time back for myself. No, it wasn't hours at a time, but even 5 minutes of being able to sit by yourself without something *needing* you felt like a break to me.

It didn't happen overnight, and it was a slow process, but eventually both my children learned how to entertain themselves without interaction from me, TV, or other kids.

Allowing your children to be bored is the best thing you can do for your babies/kids. It forces them to become self-sufficient in seeking out the right type and amount of stimulation they require. I'm not saying ignore a baby whose basic needs haven't been met. What I am saying is that it's totally fine and beneficial for your baby to be near you but not engaging with you several times during the day.

Arthur usually found/preferred a quiet place to play and think when given alone time, whereas Ivy made as much noise and caused as much destruction as she could. Kids are different and require different levels of stimulation. They know what they need, so give them the space to tell you by showing you through their actions. Observe and just try and understand what motivates your little one naturally.

How every family accomplishes this will look different. For instance, in a single-parent family home maybe the "alone" time for the child is in the morning whilst the parent gets ready for the day. But in the evening the parent has carved out space to spend quality time with their child. Remember, children thrive in structure. Knowing what happens next makes them feel safe, especially babies.

Also, keep life as simple as possible. Don't feel the need to hurry up and rush your child to grow up by exposing them to activities/stimulation that is too much for them to process. We are talking the first 2 years (730) days of their life. They don't need to see a movie, or go on a Disney cruise, or attend 5 different classes a week.

They need a stable caregiver who can provide flexibility within a daily structure of monotony with minimal to no screen time. However, if you do allow TV/screens, make sure it is active time and you are engaged in the process. Lastly, make sure to provide times for boredom when they are at their "best" (rested, fed, etc.), so they learn from a young age how to explore their world and get used to filling a little bit of their day by themselves.

Chapter 20

LOVE AS LOUD AS YOU YELL

What's Your Parenting Style?

THE TITLE OF THIS section came to me one afternoon as I was – wait for it – yelling at my kids. To be honest I don't remember why I was yelling, just that I was sick and tired of doing it. As part of the training to become a clinical psychologist I had to learn how to be the "objective observer" during interactions with clients. This was so I could not only gather useful data about what was happening in the moment, but also so I would be able to step back from the situation and see the big picture by taking emotion out of it in order to see if anything could be done behaviorally to make a family system work more smoothly.

This brings me back to my point. Yelling. It doesn't do anyone any good. It stresses out the parents, stresses out the kids and just makes home life miserable.

I was unhappy yelling at the kids for what felt like a week straight. Upon careful and focused reflection, I realized that during that week I had been preoccupied with getting the house ready for the holidays and had not been giving as much face-to-face quality time with the kids as I usually did. The next morning, I sat the kids down and explained to them why I had been yelling so much and that I recognized I had not been paying as much attention to them as I normally did, which resulted in them seeking out attention through bad behavior.

I told them I loved them very much and that I was sorry, and that I was going to try harder to not yell as much and be more "present" mentally and physically. (Remember you are always modeling behaviors for your children so let's model manners and respect.) I pretty much said it just like that. I kept it simple and honest.

Afterward I gave them both a hug and a kiss and asked if they had anything they wanted to share, which for a 19-month-old and 3-year-old is pretty much, "OK, Momma b." I then asked them if they could also try listening a little bit better as well, to which they happily agreed. Yes, things got better almost immediately. This talk validated their existence in my life and modeled the importance of self-reflection and flexibility in shifting behaviors toward becoming a better person.

Of course, small human brains aren't fully developed nor are they capable of understanding all the nuances of what I had just explained to them on the same level as you can. That is totally fine because I was going for the bigger picture.

Their overall takeaway from the experience was this: I stopped yelling as much and paid more attention to them during the day. Consequently, they listened the first or second time I asked them to do something and usually with a smile. Another and maybe more important takeaway for them is that they were reminded they are active participants in their family system.

Even today, when I find myself yelling too much at my kids, I take a step back and see what's going on with myself first, and then see how that's impacting the kids and family system. After that, I usually make personal changes, talk about the changes with whomever it may involve and then make sure the kids know they are loved loved loved and what (if anything), they can do to help.

Usually, if you're yelling a lot at your kids you aren't being as loving and cuddly and snuggly with them because you're mad, frustrated, and fed up with them. I totally get that and it's normal. I sometimes wanted to smack the smirk off their faces and not kiss it off (but I NEVER condone violence of any kind as it doesn't solve anything).

Just know that honey catches more flies than vinegar. Don't get me wrong, I'm not saying it's fine to beat your child as long as you give them lots of kisses afterward. What I am saying is that along with providing clear, firm and consistent boundaries/rules, children need to be told they are loved, need to be treated with respect and need to feel their existence within the family system is valued.

So how do you balance being a strict boundary enforcer as well as being loving and kind? If that is your goal as a parent, then your parenting style is what is called Authoritative, but wait, I'm jumping ahead of myself.

For over 75 years researchers have been looking at how parents, well, parent. Diana Baumrind, a developmental psychologist who worked with preschoolers, noted that children responded to their parents differently, and it directly related to the parenting style of each parent. The parenting style construct commonly used in psychology today is based off of her research. I will briefly go over each parenting style she identified.

Authoritative Parenting
<u>High Expectations, High Responsiveness</u>
(considered the best approach)
These parents have high expectations for achievement and maturity when it comes to their children. Authoritative parents are the ones that love as loud as they yell. They provide firm and consistent boundaries/rules and are often very warm, loving, affectionate, supportive, and they encourage independence. Most importantly, these parents are responsive to the needs of their children. Parents have open discussions about rules and use reason and logic when it comes to consequences for both good and bad behavior. They take into account their child's feelings and opinions. Based on research, children of authoritative parents tend to be:
◊ happy and content
◊ more independent
◊ achieve higher academic success

◊ develop a good sense of self/self-esteem

◊ more competent when it comes to social skills

◊ overall exhibit less depression, anxiety, suicide attempts, delinquency, alcohol and drug use

◊ display less violent tendencies

Authoritarian Parenting

High Expectations, Low Responsiveness

I know the name of this style of parenting looks almost identical to the previous one, but I assure you it is not. Whilst their names are similar the approach is very different. The main differences between these two styles of parenting are simple, but important to note. Authoritarian parents demand blind obedience, are unresponsive to the needs of their children and in general aren't as nurturing. You know, the ones that say, "Do it because I said so." Even though Authoritative and Authoritarian parenting styles both have high standards for their children, authoritarian parents often use stern discipline (think wooden spoon spanking, kneeling on rice, mouth washed out with soap) and often employ punishment to control children's behavior. Children of authoritarian parents tend to:

◊ have an unhappy disposition

◊ exhibit less independence

◊ display insecurities

◊ have lower self-esteem

◊ display more behavioral problems

◊ perform poorly in school

◊ underdeveloped social skills

◊ often more prone to mental issues

Permissive Parenting (Indulgent)

Low Expectations, High Responsiveness

These are the parents most kids think they want. You know, the parents that set very few rules and boundaries and rarely enforce them. These parents are often perceived by children as fun, warm, rarely say "no" and never want to be perceived as the "bad guy". Children of permissive parents tend to:

◊   struggle following rules

◊   display underdeveloped self-control

◊   exhibit egocentric tendencies

◊   Because they think they are the center of the world they struggle to maintain relationships and display underdeveloped social interactions

Neglectful Parenting (Uninvolved)

Low Expectations, Low responsiveness

Parents who are uninvolved in their children's lives and who do not set boundaries and expect little to nothing from their children are labeled as Neglectful parents.

Extreme cases are the ones we see on the news which talk about a parent who left their 5 and 3 year-old home for the weekend. Uninvolved parents tend to also suffer from one or more of the following: mental health issues, had mothers who suffered from severe depression, experienced childhood neglect, and/or survivors of physical/sexual/emotional abuse. Often, these types of parents suffer from a combination of the above problems and their family genogram is full of similar stories. Children of neglectful parents tend to be:

◊   more impulsive

◊   underdeveloped ability to self-regulate emotions

◊   in trouble with authority figures/law

◊   suffer from mental health issues

Authoritative parenting is widely regarded as the most effective and beneficial parenting style. But just like in life, there are always exceptions to the rules. It's important to note how cultural and ethnic differences impact parenting. In non-Caucasian families, studies found that authoritative parenting wasn't always linked to the best school achievement.

One study found that even when African-American students had authoritative parents, if the student did not have peer support, they under-performed academically. Another study showed that Asian-American students performed the best in school when they had authoritarian parents and peer support. And the last study I will share was done in Spain where both indulgent and authoritative parenting styles were associated with good outcomes. Keep in mind these studies only compared school performance and parenting styles. Not the child's overall emotional well-being.

My style of parenting is Authoritative, if you hadn't guessed already. I have very high expectations for my children but use humor, fun, love and firm boundaries to get results. Oh, yelling, don't forget that one. Yelling is the easiest way to get results, but the results don't stick, and your children are minding you out of fear. So how can you get results without yelling?

Let me give you an example using my kids. First, I'm gonna hit you with the short of it. I let my 11-month-old little girl cry off and on for 45 minutes at the bottom of a staircase whilst I sat on another floor with her older brother watching TV. That's cold-blooded, I know. But now I'm gonna give you the long of it.

I rarely let the kids watch TV and the three of us were headed upstairs to watch *Winnie the Pooh* as a special treat, and Ivy had picked the show. Ivy had started walking around 10 months and could easily crawl upstairs. My hands were full with a tray of yummy snacks and when we got to the stairs Ivy wanted to be carried. I told her politely that I couldn't carry her because I was carrying her snacks, but if she moved her little bum upstairs, we would watch the show *she* had chosen.

She proceeded to pout and throw a small tantrum to which I replied, "I don't mind if you cry it's not going to make me pick you up. Ivy, we are going upstairs to start the show. If you want to watch it with us, come upstairs."

Arthur and I went upstairs and started the show. Throughout the show she would cry on and off depending on if she wanted my attention or not, and we all know those cries... you know, the ones when you start whispering and the kid immediately stops crying so they can hear what you're saying.

I could easily see her sitting at the bottom of the stairs and checked on her every few minutes when she was quiet (she couldn't see me from the angle I was looking). I even went downstairs on two separate occasions to "wash my hands" and ask Ivy if I could hold her hand as she walked upstairs. She refused and would start screaming again. I would just turn around and go back into the attic where we were watching TV.

With about 10 minutes left in the show, I noticed Ivy had quietly crawled up the stairs and was happily smiling as she waddled to the sofa to sit between her brother and myself and watched the last few minutes. Then we turned the TV off and the kids played.

I gave a reasonable request. I knew she could easily complete the task. She refused. I didn't cave in to her demands, and I provided opportunities to help her make the right choice. And at the end of the day, as it is with every child, we as parents have to give them enough space to make decisions on their own in their *own time,* even at 11 months old.

I didn't just leave her alone unsupervised in a dangerous location for 45 minutes and for no reason. I didn't demand she go upstairs. I remained calm and in control. This was our first ever standoff and I *had* to win. Dude, after leaving her downstairs for 20 minutes I had to be committed to this, or else any future standoff would be even worse because each time you cave, you are resetting the "bar" for just how awful they have to be before you give them what they want.

I sure wasn't planning on listening to an 11-month-old mad-scream/cry for another 20 minutes anytime soon. That's why I don't set a line very often, or if I do, I try to be rational and calm about it and know I will be able to follow through with whatever consequence I set.

Anyway, I told my partner as soon as she got home from work what had happened, and we laughed and laughed. We both are dreading the teenage years.

Chapter 21

I'M NOT QUESTIONING YOU; I AM GATHERING DATA
Communicating Effectively with Your Co-Parent

MY PARTNER IS THE Yin to my Yang, the salt to my pepper, the hip to my hop, the tick to my tock and at times the biggest pain in my neck. We work so well together because our differences and similarities are often mirror images of each other, thereby creating the ideal balance.

Early in our relationship we discovered that our arguments often stemmed from the fact that we simply view the world differently, neither vantage point being right or wrong, and we usually ended up agreeing on the outcome of whatever started the discussion/argument.

She is awesome at her job because she chose a career she is naturally good at... finding potential problems and fixing them before they spiral out of control (her degree is in accounting, she's a numbers person). I too chose a career I'm naturally inclined toward, which is interacting with others and using my natural positive energy/outlook toward life and my "nothing can stop us" attitude to help inspire people to live truer, more fulfilling and satisfying lives.

For me, my natural tendency is to leap before I look, and once I land to figure out the next step. This approach in life has worked for me. My partner's natural tendency is to calculate the approximate speed she will need to reach her destination and research the weather conditions to assess for any potential elements of surprise (wind, rain, etc.).

Then she would compute where she would land and what she will do after she does. Following that she would sleep on this plan and make her final decision the following morning. Yes, of course I am over-exaggerating to make a point, but you get my drift, right? Most of the time she and I land at the same spot but if it's not exactly the same we are usually close to each other and make a compromised decision from a place of respect and love. I leap and live and she plans and prevails.

Our relationship (the dynamic of the Yin and Yang), will resonate with many of you, and for those that it doesn't, wonderful! You and your partner communicate and see the world from a similar lens; that's not to say you won't have disagreements, because you will. Everyone disagrees with someone at some point in their life, and that's normal and healthy and natural. The issues arise when a dyad (the couple), are unable to speak respectfully to one another and therefore are unable to come to an agreement that both will be able to live with.

One way around this type of interaction is to create boundaries wherein one person makes all the decisions about X and the other makes all the decisions about Y. When it comes to parenting, I often saw this arrangement with couples who both held very traditional roles in the home. One parent would make all the decisions about the kids/house and the other person made all the decisions about the money and big spending items like purchasing the house, car etc. The couple did this because they found that easier than having to work through disagreements and come to compromises together.

Both sides have their pros and cons, just try to figure out what type of relationship you have with your partner and ask yourself if you like it and is it working for you and your family. Just so you know, research shows that the couples who work things out have the stronger foundation for coping with blows to the dyad (infidelity, death of a child), than couples who keep things "calm" on the surface but are drowning underwater in unsaid complaints and frustrations with their partner.

Along with having a check-in with yourself (and partner), about how you guys resolve disagreements, it's important to know your own (and their), language of love. Cause once a baby arrives in your lives you become so exhausted and in need of emotional support that knowing "just what to do" will be important, valuable and helpful in keeping peace at a time of intense stress on the couple.

The idea of people having different languages of love is a concept developed and written by Dr. Chapman. Essentially, a language of love is the way a person speaks, shows, and understands emotional love. A lot has been written about how you show love and how you prefer/need others to show you their love. I won't go into great detail, but here is the list with a brief description of the different love languages:

1. *Words of Affirmation* – Saying things like "You look great" or "You are amazing, and I love you" or "Thanks for trying so hard and being such an amazing parent to our children."
2. *Acts of Service* – Doing things for this person like helping out with the dishes even if it isn't your night.
3. *Receiving Gifts* – No, this doesn't mean the person is materialistic; it's not about the amount of money of the gift it's the fact you thought about them. Even a bouquet of dandelions presented in a nice way could be meaningful. It's the thought that counts.
4. *Quality Time* – Spending time with someone without distractions of TV, phones, etc. They want your undivided attention and need to feel as though they are the main event.
5. *Physical Touch* – Nothing is more impactful than physical touch and no number of gifts or words can make up for hugs, cuddles, holding hands, etc. (no, this isn't about sex).

When I read the above list, I think WTF I want *all* of it! Gifts, rub my feet, do the dishes and definitely tell me how bloody fabulous I look with my upswept hair, smelly-baby-puke stained t-shirt, and oh so baggy sweatpants which are in fact 5 sizes too big for me so I at least can feel "skinny" in one pair of pants for one day a week.

You get my drift; just know there should be one of those languages of love that makes you feel loved more than the others. Learn about both you and your partner's language of love because when you're both exhausted knowing how to make each other happy by doing a little bit can go a long way.

All in all, my partner and I work well together. It's those times when we are both feeling overwhelmed, tired and emotionally drained that communication with one another gets messed up. It's like I have a line of adolescent teens in my head playing the old game "telephone" but messing up the message as it travels, just to be jerks. So when my partner says, "Where is the pacifier?" I sometimes would hear, "You are the most incompetent person I have ever met. I can't believe you are in charge of these small people every day and they are still alive – where is the pacifier?" Yup, some days are just like that.

Remember to be kind to each other and respect each other. It's so so easy to fall into a pattern of interacting with your partner that is disrespectful and hurtful to one another. It can happen quickly and without the two of you even being aware of it. Figure out your language of love and your partner's. Talk about it with them and maybe even give each other advice or ideas on what they could do when you are feeling blue. If they speak a different language of love, they may not have a clue how to make you feel loved, so just tell them. Have patience with one another. Remember this time when your babies are young and you're exhausted won't last forever.

Chapter 22

SEX DRIVE

The Tank is on Empty but I Appreciate Your Wax Job

WHEN I STARTED MY doctorate program in Clinical Psychology, I quit my full-time job as a music therapist, bought a condo on Chicago's south side (51st and Martin Luther King Drive to be precise), and started looking for part-time work where I could maximize both time and potential earnings.

As it happened, I found a job running a not-for-profit, which provides free exercise opportunities for children with disabilities (Kids Enjoy Exercise Now: KEEN). I was the only part-time paid staff member and my job was to both manage a pool of volunteers (around 700 in the database when I left the job) and grow programs. I was to report to a board of directors, and the board's president was essentially my boss. She asked me to meet each board member when I joined the team to introduce myself and get to know them a little. I reached out to everyone and the last person I was to meet with was the board treasurer.

Via email, she (the treasurer), and I decided to meet at a restaurant and I was running late. As I searched for parking, my eyes were drawn to a beautiful, confident and striking woman walking past the meeting place and I thought to myself, "Why couldn't *she* have been the person I was coming to meet?"

As the story goes, that woman *was* the treasurer (she had missed the restaurant). That gorgeous, confident, timeless beauty was there to meet me!

After we knew each other a bit more she admitted to having a similar experience of instant connection to me when I had stepped into the restaurant. Needless to say, the attraction was immediate for both of us *even* before we knew each other.

The treasurer ended up being my current and only partner. She is stunning, confident, tall, athletic and feminine in a classic/timeless kind of way. I adore her with all my heart, mind, body and soul.

The feeling is mutual. She knows me so well she once told me this metaphor about how she sees us (she knows I love metaphors).

She views me as a wild horse that lives in the mountains near the edges of a flat, lush, peaceful meadow/ranch. She is the proud owner of this ranch and works very hard to make it beautiful. Even after I commit to living with her on her peaceful and orderly ranch, she knows there is one thing she can never do. She can never put up a fence and expect me to calmly and happily stay put. As Sinatra sang so well, "Don't fence me in." She knows not to put up a fence and I know to not run far from home, and it works for both of us.

God, I adore her. So, when I started taking hormone pills a year before I got pregnant, I noticed my sexual desire started to wane. Then after I got pregnant, I unfortunately was *not* one of those women who get really horny.

I share with you that back-story because it lets you know just how deep my attraction to my partner is and how hard it was living with and loving someone, but not wanting to touch or be touched sexually by them after having children.

This isn't uncommon, losing one's sex drive after a baby arrives. You're tired, feeling incompetent as a parent because this is all new to you, your body (if you had the baby), is undergoing crazy amounts of hormonal changes, and if you didn't have a baby, you too are suffering from a catastrophic disruption to your life.

Everyone I spoke to and everything I've read said it's not

uncommon for couples to experience a decrease in intimacy after a baby arrives. Life is chaotic and new parents are merely trying to find their footing in the quicksand that is the learning curve of parenting.

When the kids were 9 months and 28 months old, we had just returned from Christmas with family in the UK (international travel, sleep-deprived parents and kids who wouldn't nap made the visit quite stressful), and my partner and I desperately needed a date night. A movie that we had been waiting a year to see due to delayed release dates was finally in the theaters. So we found a babysitter and went to the matinee.

The movie was called *Carol* and the storyline is about two women in the 1950s who fall in love and struggle to come to terms with their sexuality, and also cope with society's limits on a lesbian couple. There is only one sex scene and even then, it's nothing raunchy. Nevertheless, the innocence, intimacy, and the sheer desire that I saw between the actresses was enough to make the area below my belt start to tingle again.

Yup you heard me correctly, tingle. Like when your foot falls asleep due to lack of blood flow. I was sooooo excited to feel those sensations again after 3 ½ years that I paid a babysitter to watch the children on 4 different occasions during a week's time frame so I could see the show over and over again to try and prime the pump.

You know, it's like after winter when you get the lawn mower out to cut the grass for the first time in spring. Right after you've added fresh gasoline you hit the squishy button, pump, pump, pump, pump and force that gasoline down those dry tubes to get the juice where it needs to be so that the bloody thing can start. That kinda pumping.

Carol the movie was it for me. To stay with the engine metaphor, that movie replaced my old, worn out spark plug, and seeing the show over and over helped my body wake up. Now, it was time to focus on tuning up the rest of my engine.

No, the movie wasn't a panacea that suddenly fixed everything and put my sex drive back where it used to be. But it did provide the missing element that was needed to remind me I am a sexual being and there are parts of my body that have been asleep for a long, long time.

Besides seeing the movie and consciously thinking about sex (or lack thereof), what also helped was talking about and being open with my partner about what I was/wasn't feeling sexually. My mind wanted it (if for nothing else than exercise reasons), but I just couldn't get my head around it.

It wasn't just the physical aspect of not having a high sex drive, I also struggled with the mental aspect of turning off my brain long enough to "get in the mood". A thousand things race through my mind normally, but add in the feeding, sleeping, pooping, burping schedules of two more humans and you're lucky if I remember your name.

There were so many thoughts, including: *"Why am I not horny and how can I get horny? How can I increase my sex drive? Will my boobs always be this big and sensitive? Did I give the dogs their pills? Do I think Ivy's diaper rash will be better in the morning? When do I need to redo my credits for my professional license? God, my ass and thighs are huge. What should I cook for dinner tomorrow night?"* You get my drift. It was mentally and physically hard for me to get in the mood after having kids.

Some couples are lucky and never run into issues in the sack. Unfortunately, that wasn't me. Regardless of how non-existent my sex drive was, I always saw my partner as beautiful, caring, sensual and attractive. She maintained her "wax job" both on the outside *and* inside. Always beautiful and always supportive… she just waited patiently for me to figure myself out.

If you're the person who wants more sex, just know that patience is sexy to someone struggling to find his or her mojo. Talking about your lack of sex drive can help and trying to reconnect to your earlier years of horniness can help, too. Try not to focus too much on it and recognize that you are not alone in your struggle to get your motor running. Lastly, if nothing seems to be helping remember sex therapists exist and help couples all the time figure out how to make their relationships stronger through sexual intimacy.

SECTION III

Last But NOT Least

Chapter 23

HISTORY REPEATS ITSELF; BUT IT DOESN'T HAVE TO
To Change our Future We Must First Explore our Past

I BET YOU WOULD agree with me that at some (or many), points in your life you've said, "I will never grow up and be like my parents!" – and BAM! – you find yourself doing the same things and saying the exact same phrases you swore you *never* would say to your kids.

Most things in life follow a pattern or specific way of doing/being. Often these repetitions/patterns happen for a specific reason. Looking at things from an anthropological perspective, traditions are important for humans to feel connected to a specific place and to people that we call home. Another example is the survival of a species. If a baby doesn't suckle for milk, it will starve and those genes will not be passed on.

Or, we don't have to have a good reason, such as why great great great Grandma's fruitcake recipe is used instead of a tastier, new recipe for a holiday dessert. "Well, that's just how we do it in this house," (or your family's version of that), is thrown in your face and so the pattern continues.

It continues because humans are genetically coded to connect socially; we seek out companions and feel "in sync" when those around us do similar or the same things as us. This ensures the survival of our species. Don't get me wrong, there is always that one "dark horse/black sheep" of the family that embraces not "fitting in", but for the most part everyone wants to be liked and understood by others, especially one's family.

We humans have always been social creatures whose interpersonal relationships have evolved throughout hundreds of thousands of years. The physical changes of our early ancestors called hominids directly impacted how the males and females related to each other. Once hominids had learned to walk on two feet and the size/strength of the sexes became more equitable (i.e. females could physically resist unwanted sexual intercourse from men in the group), males were forced to come up with "new ways" to gain the interest of the opposite sex in an effort to mate.

Consequently, those males who were not blessed with physical attractiveness developed other skills like singing and dancing to attract mates. Think of famous male musicians, how many can you name that has the frame of a footballer and the looks of Brad Pitt? Not many. Instead brilliant men like Prince and Paul Simon pop into my mind, and they were both small in stature. But I doubt they ever wanted for "mates".

The change in physical stature meant a change in how males and females had to relate to each other on an emotional level. A law in physics states that to every action we take an equal and opposite reaction will occur. It's not that hard to surmise that relationships between the sexes of our early ancestors definitely had some emotional kinks to work out once the women were able to say, "Nope, not tonight, you big hairy ape."

Just as families today, members of those early family units had specific roles to fulfill to ensure the survival of the group. I'm not talking just about who collects the water and who picks berries; I'm referring to the emotional roles we take on in our family.

One psychologist, Dr. Murray Bowen, believed that individuals couldn't be understood in isolation from one another, but rather as a part of their family. He (and I), believe families are systems of interconnected and interdependent individuals, none of whom can be understood in isolation from the system.

The number of times a parent would drop off their "naughty kid" for therapy and expect me to "fix" their child having only spent 45 minutes a week with them was ridiculously high, and I would tell them it was an insane idea to expect such outcomes. No one lives in a vacuum. Your life and actions impact everyone else around you. Understanding your own family's patterns of interacting and communicating can make you a more aware and present parent.

Which brings me to my point: you don't have to "become" your parents *if* you take time to identify/understand your own family patterns of interactions and relationships and make a conscious effort to change them.

Take a minute and imagine your family as a system/machine in which each member has a role to play and rules to respect. Within your family I'm sure there were/are certain expectations of how you interact with family members, like not talking back to your parents. Every member of your family is expected to respond to each other in a certain way, according to the role they inherited.

For example, one of the roles I play in my family is the "oddball". I *love* this role because it gives me freedom and space to be weird, but it also means I sometimes feel ostracized and lonely. Out of all my cousins (there are 7 of us, not small but not huge) I am the only person who doesn't identify as straight. It's a little ironic to me, and a nod to my parents for normalizing adoption so much, that I never thought I was "odd" due to the fact that I was adopted. Of course, having a sister and dad who were also adopted helped to normalize it, but I never felt that aspect was what made me different from the rest of my family.

This one time, one of my aunts told a group of family members that she knew I was adopted because, "No one with our family blood would be gay." I wasn't present, but two cousins confirmed she did say it. At the time I had just come out to my family after 28 years of trying SOOOO hard to force myself to be somebody I wasn't. It didn't feel great, but it merely confirmed, "Yup, you're different and that's fine."

What is your role in the family? Are you the emotional caretaker of everyone or maybe the whipping "person" whom everyone takes his or her frustration out on, or maybe both? Are you the rock of the family? The person that isn't allowed to be vulnerable or weak because if you show weakness or fear, the rest of the family who lean on you emotionally suddenly panic and freak out. Or maybe you're the victim of the family. Always sick, always in a crisis, and the rallying around your hot mess is what brings the family together, which keeps you being a hot mess. See how the cycle goes?

Along with understanding the specific role you play in your family, gaining a broader view (genogram) of familial patterns of interpersonal relationships can also be helpful. A genogram provides a visual representation of the personalities and the interplay of generations within a family. It can also be used to identify repetitive patterns of behavior and medical conditions; it's a psychological family tree, if you will.

I remember working with a seven-year-old girl who had been sexually molested by her cousin. During the first few sessions, her mother was involved and provided family history for a genogram. The mother wept as she realized the history of sexual/emotional/physical abuse the women in her family had endured at the hands of men/fathers, uncles, brothers and cousins in her family tree.

During this time it came to light that a cousin had sexually abused the mother when she was 10 years old. The little girl held her mother, stroked her hair and whispered to her, "It's going to be okay, Mom. It's going to be okay." That moment was bittersweet for me because I ached for that little 7-year-old girl who was thrust into the role of "comforter/rock" and raped of both physical and emotional innocence. I also felt deeply for this mother who wanted to break the "shitty cycle" and was the first in her family to seek out therapy for herself and daughter. Awareness is the first step in changing a pattern of behavior and action must follow.

Understanding yourself is one of the best presents you can give your partner, your children, and the world in general, really. Take the time to do your own family tree and if you feel so inclined, go seek out a therapist. No shame in knowing more about yourself and how your family role and styles of communication impact who you are and your parenting. I know that many of the women in my family tend to be passive-aggressive in how they communicate their feelings and often are unable to provide a compliment without also adding 2 digs at the same time, "just to make sure you don't get too full of yourself."

For example, at my doctoral graduation I was introducing my family to the Clinical Training Director and close mentor at my school. He was telling my family that they must be proud of all my hard work and my mother classically responds, "Oh, well, she will always just be Bethany to us, not Doctor." I was gutted. Jesus, Mom! I have just taken out hundreds of thousands of dollars in loans, spent thousands of hours studying, writing, and working with people for 6 ½ years, not to mention the social sacrifices I had to make to create time to do all the schoolwork. Couldn't she have just said, "Yes, we are proud"?

Regardless, a comment like that was expected. In my family we don't want anyone thinking that they are somehow better than anyone else. Keep the status quo. No joke, once an elder in my family said that when she disagreed with another family member it was because they just had "…too much education."

Please don't get me wrong, I'm not judging my family. I'm merely pointing out this unspoken rule of communication that keeps getting passed through each generation in my family tree. I just want you to think about your family and some of the unspoken rules of communication you have.

Let me give you another unspoken rule about my family that I think others may be able to relate to and it even ties into my previous example. After a post-graduation celebration lunch with my family I took my mother aside and asked her why she said what she did to my professor. This is kinda how the conversation went.

ME: *Mom, I was wondering why you said what you did to my prof when he was essentially giving you a compliment as a parent by saying how "nicely" I turned out.*

MOM: *What did I say wrong? I said we would never call you doctor? What's wrong with that?...* (Wait for it... this is the comment that I'm sure many of you have heard before.) *I'm sorry you heard it that way.*

Oh, snap, no she didn't! Did you think that was an apology? That's her saying she feels sorry for me that I got upset. Not that she is sorry for what she said.

In my family, compliments are usually laced with venom and spite and try as you might... you will never get a simple "I'm sorry". If you did, that would be seen as a sign of weakness and we can never be weak in our family. Sound familiar? Maybe your version is not quite exactly the same, but similar? You can't show weakness? What happens if you do? Family rules can be spoken and unspoken.

Along with not being able to show mental weakness in my family, you can't be physically weak either. Once, I overheard one of my aunts and a great aunt both complaining about how my cousins were raising their kids and how "outside influences" (spouses) were to be blamed.

I asked what they were talking about. Apparently, when their grandkids (who range in age from 18 months – 8 years), fall down, the aunts get annoyed when they hear, "Are you OK to get up?" compared to what I heard my entire childhood, which was, "Get up, you're okay," and if you didn't stop crying quickly enough it was followed up by a, "I'll give you something to cry about."

The same words put in a different order make the meaning of the phrase completely different:

"Get up! You're okay!" Vs. "Are you okay to get up?"

How do you know if your little newly walking 14-month-old is OK or not? How come you get to be judge of how they feel? I wasn't given the choice and "told" from a young age that what I was emotionally feeling wasn't accurate and I needed to just toughen up. Yes, it has made me very strong, but the other side of the sword is I don't ask for help when I need to and I struggle to cry for my own pain and sorrow. Pick your poison.

Growing up I really hated always feeling like I had to defend myself, my choices and my decisions if they varied at all from the strict guidelines my family and religion had for me. Looking for faults in others is something that comes easily to me; nevertheless, I wanted to break this pattern of communication. Therefore, I've worked hard, in and out of therapy, since I was 18 years old to hold up a mirror to myself and look at the good, bad, and the ugly in order to change.

One of the things I changed was the passive-aggressive communication style many use in my family. I am now quite direct in my communication with everyone, even family members (who are still getting used to it). For instance, one of my grandmas was going on and on and on about the amount of effort and time I was putting into making sandwiches for everyone for lunch. I was getting irritated at what I perceived to be constant badgering and so I kindly but directly said,

"Hey, Gram, as you know I love to cook so I am putting a lot of effort into this sandwich, so every bite is the 'perfect' bite. But I tell you what. If after you have a few bites and it's not the best sandwich you've eaten in a long time you just tell me, and the next time you all come up I will happily order pizza."

Yes, everyone in the room was quiet because no one knew what to say. My family isn't used to direct, honest, straightforward communication. Also, I am pretty sure my grandma wasn't trying to be mean and annoying; she more than likely was struggling with the feeling of loss about *her* family role.

As the youngest and only girl of 6 siblings, my grandma shared with me that at a young age she was told her role in the family was to be in the kitchen cooking for the men who worked the farm. I imagine it was hard for my grandma to watch someone stepping into the role she had filled since she was a little girl.

In the moment, I wasn't able to see how my grandma's passive-aggressive banter was probably her trying to be a part of the preparation of the meal. Or maybe she felt like a burden and didn't like the idea of someone caring for her. I don't know the answer. So, I picked a possible reason that makes me feel the best and moved on. Oh, and yes, *everyone* complimented me on how good the sandwiches were.

Family roles don't always stay the same. Just as my grandma used to be the one who cooked and fed everyone, now she is the one being cared for and there is a huge loss of independence that I'm sure she is struggling to cope with. Other examples of when family roles change could be that a new baby pushes the old baby into the role of "big" sibling. Another time could be if the primary breadwinner of the family is no longer able to work and roles switch for the parents.

Every time a role shifts within a family unit, everyone will be impacted by it directly or indirectly. Be aware of the change and try to be a bit more understanding as people re-adjust in your family unit.

Lastly, please don't feel overwhelmed with all of the information I am throwing your way. I simply want to plant some seeds in your mind of different things to think about when raising your children, and just maybe those seeds may grow roots and choose to bloom. If you don't like therapy and you don't want to go, don't go. But at least ponder about your family role and unspoken family rules that you may not want to pass on to your kids.

May we raise kinder, gentler people and change the world one kid at a time. All the things I mention in this section aren't easily identifiable, especially by one's self. They say we can't see the forest when we are standing amongst the trees. However, through work in therapy and/or self-reflection, one can begin to unravel old patterns of interaction and develop healthier ways to communicate.

Becoming aware of your own familial patterns of relating to each other and how that impacts you and your parenting is something I think every new parent should consider. What kind of parent do you want to be? My mom told me many times, usually when I was complaining about her parenting skills, to take the things she did well and make them even better. And then take the things she wasn't doing great and change it. Sound advice, Mom, I'm taking it.

Chapter 24

NURTURE VS. NATURE AND TEMPERAMENT
We Are All Born with a Specific Temperament. How Does Our Environment Shape Us?

THE FIRST 9 MONTHS of my life were not the best; I had been physically neglected, lived with my biological mother/aunt/grandmother, had been in and out of seven foster homes, adopted, and returned all *before* my parents adopted me.

So, yeah… I had/have attachment issues.

From the first day my parents brought me home, my mother told me I never really bonded with her. I wouldn't let her hold me or cuddle me unless I was in physical pain, and only then would I let her rock me in a chair. The social workers thought the lack of attachment to my mother was because I had been neglected and abused by females during the first 9 months of my life.

I loved being around men: all men, my dad, and even strange men in the grocery stores. I say that because my mom told me once that I was having a full-blown meltdown at a store and she tried to pick me up off the floor because I was kicking and screaming, and I went "spaghetti" on her (you know… how kids can suddenly go limp?). So, she asked a strange man walking by if he could pick me up. The minute he did I stopped crying and just "hung out" in his arms for a bit whilst my mom paid for her groceries.

It was a funny story to hear told over and over as a child and at many multi-generational family gatherings. Everyone would laugh and laugh at the stories my mom and dad told about my "fits".

As a child, when I got upset I used to lie on the floor and kick my heels together until they bled. My parents tried everything to stop these fits. My pediatrician even recommended throwing a glass of water on me or lying next to me on the floor and throwing a fit, too. My mom said she tried both suggestions and I did stop for a second as I stared at her as if she had completely lost the plot.

Alas, nothing really helped except time and maturity. At some point when I was around 11 or 12 years old, I eventually stopped throwing tantrums. By that point in my life I knew that throwing a fit wouldn't get me what I wanted so self-control (ego) became stronger than impulses (id).

Knowing what I know about the importance of attachment and consistency in forming early bonds with babies, I always figured my lack of attachment to the females in my family was simply due to the abuse from females prior to my adoption. Research has also confirmed this idea; one's early relationships with their primary caregiver and immediate family/caregivers are what lay the foundation for all future relationships. I'm talking not only psychologically but also neurologically. Remember the section on how touching a baby actually helps wire their brain?

Because Ivy did not bond with my partner until she was around 12 months old, I was forced to revisit the idea that maybe my attachment issues weren't solely due to my early relationships/environment but rather had a deeper genetic component.

This genetic component is what psychologists call temperament. Things such as eye color, hair color and even temperament are wired the minute the egg and sperm meet and are considered to be determined by DNA. Other things such as weight and height have genetic components to them but can be altered by one's environment/nature. For example, even if you have the genes to be 6'8", if you aren't provided the right kind of diet at a young age your body won't grow to its fullest potential.

So, what does this mean? I was born not wanting to bond with my mom due to my temperament? Enter the debate of Nature vs. Nurture. Essentially the debate is about whether human behavior is solely determined by the environment (this includes pre-natal), or by a person's genes (DNA).

It's hard for me to imagine that any baby given the right environmental exposures could become anything they wanted. Let's say for argument's sake two babies were taken from birth and both exposed to music and given extensive and intensive music lessons from a young age. You would expect them to both have the same skill level but it just doesn't work that way.

I'm sure you know families where one of the children is gifted in sports or music but the others aren't? One could argue all the siblings were exposed to the same parent(s)/opportunities but why did one child excel? More than likely it is the combination of natural gifts (talent), internally motivated desire to keep practicing (temperament) and a supportive environment (nurture).

Take any one of those elements away and the kid probably wouldn't be as successful. We all know people who have a natural talent but they don't have the self-discipline/desire to do anything with it, and I'm not just talking about sports or music. Someone's ability could be that of a natural born leader (temperament), who relies on their environment (nature), to guide them toward what they will do with this skill. Will they lead a gang of thugs or will they start a movement that will change the world for the better?

A psychological definition of temperament is a set of inborn traits that organize an individual's approach to the world. You know, have you always seen the glass as half full or half empty? Are you naturally optimistic or pessimistic in your approach to things in life? It's important to know that these traits are relatively stable from birth. We've all heard someone say "…that baby is so good natured," or "...that baby's got the devil in him." (Obviously most people don't share the last comment with the parents but save it for friends and distant relatives.)

Remember, temperament is genetic and temperament traits play a vital role in the development of your child's distinct personality. They also determine how your little one learns about the world around them. Do they leap and live or plan and prevail?

The good news is that temperament is genetic, so you might get a mini version of yourself. The bad news is that temperament is genetic, so you might get a mini version of yourself. It's a double-edged sword. Yes, you will have a greater understanding and capacity for more empathy toward your child if you share the same temperament, but the likelihood that ya'll butt heads is hella high; I ain't gonna lie.

This brings me back to my little girl Ivy. According to the people who know both Ivy and me, we are like two peas in a pod, the exact same in temperament. My son Arthur has the temperament of my partner, who also shares the same temperament of donor dad (yes, this was a conscious choice). Arthur and my partner are mainly rational, cautious, kind, calm thinkers who enjoy problem solving and fixing things. Ivy was blessed (or cursed), with my temperament: strong-willed, fearless, and determined.

Both she and I have to work harder at being kind, and we are naturally inclined to show affection for others through more aggressive actions like shoving, hitting, and pinching. No don't worry; I no longer go around punching people I want to befriend; I use my words instead. For example, I had a mate in college tell me she knew she was my friend the day I saw her in the hall and cried out to her, "What's up, bitch!" She had never been happier in her life to be called bitch because she knew that me calling her that meant I really liked her... and we laughed about that!

That old saying "boys will be boys" is the biggest load of hogwash I have ever heard. It's simply not true and often used as an excuse when little boys behave badly or act out physically. My daughter would totally fit the above expression but since she's a girl she gets labeled "tomboy".

Interestingly, it seems girls have been acting like "boys" since the 1570s when the word *tomboy* was first recorded and defined as a "bold or immodest woman" or that of "a girl who acts like a spirited boy", which was recorded in the 1590s. Maybe it's about time for people to start seeing children as their own unique person instead of trying to label them as "this way" or "that way". Both boys and girls may have a tendency to show emotionality and affection through rough physical contact.

I've worked really hard throughout my life to curb my impulsive desires to run and jump on someone's back, or when having a good back and forth with a mate I want to excitedly touch them which turns into a shove (don't know my own strength) and then someone gets hurt.

My little girl is exactly the same way. She loves people and is energized by them (extrovert), but when meeting new friends, she sometimes will just walk up to them and shove them down. Of course, I tell her to apologize and try to give her words or other actions she could use to let someone know she likes them. She just wants their attention and to play with them. I know this because I see it in her behavior, but I also recall as a child doing the same things.

When I was young my mom gave me a badge that said, "HERE COMES TROUBLE" and I proudly wore that badge for years. It was another "role" I filled, and a role that I was able to pull myself out of when I got older. Remember, when you put a label on your child, be careful because it just might stick.

At the end of the day I believe nature (genetics) accounts for more than nurture (environment). When it comes to understanding yourself and what makes you tick, knowing yourself will help you know your child. If you don't know your temperament you can go online and take the Keirsey Temperament Sorter. Even if you are raising a non-biological child, knowledge is power and by understanding yourself you will be able to better understand your children thereby meeting their needs in the most effective way for both of you.

Chapter 25

LOSS OF IDENTITY
Going from Dr. Cook to Momma B

FROM THE TIME I started kindergarten at age 5 until I graduated with my doctorate degree at age 33, I spent all but 2 years in some sort of formal education setting. My identity for most of my life was a student. Then finally, after years and years of hard work, struggle, and perseverance, I achieved the highest honor awarded to someone in academia, the title of doctor.

No, I am not the type of person who throws that title around and I prefer that people don't initially know my educational background. To be honest, telling someone I'm a psychologist either shuts them up immediately or I get asked my opinion on a "tiny" issue. Up until the time Arthur was born, I was a happy, pregnant doctor doing my rounds at the rehabilitation hospitals, testing clients, and feeling pretty proud of my accomplishments in life. Then 2 weeks before he was born, I stopped being seen as Dr. Cook, but instead became the pregnant lady waiting to have her baby. I was lounging around the house, feeling fat and bloated as a cow, and struggling to breathe as the baby pushed on every organ in my body.

Just like that, I went from a title that I worked my ass off for most of my life to achieve to a title that can be given to "any woman" willing to care for a child (totally irrational thought, I know). It felt to me like the title "mother" was something that you didn't have to work very hard to achieve and therefore I viewed it as less than.

After Arthur's birth I found it very difficult to answer the question, "Are you or will you be going back to work?" As if staying home full-time with a baby isn't work! Yes, I knew what they meant, but the question in and of itself devalues the notion or idea that parenthood is less valuable than a paycheck.

Finding your footing after a baby arrives and rocks your world, is not always easy. For the first year of Arthur's life I spoke countless times with my partner about how I was feeling "less than" because I wasn't bringing home money and didn't feel I had a true identity anymore. She kindly listened, validated, and kept reinforcing the idea that I was doing the most important job in the world by raising our children.

She could have told me that every day multiple times a day, and I still wouldn't have been able to break that annoying inner-voice-tape-loop that played in my brain. You know, the one that says you'll never be good enough, smart enough, fast enough, rich enough etc.? Or at least, mine says that.

After I became a mother, I began to appreciate just how judgmental I actually was about other people and their parenting. It was only through recognizing my own bias toward mothers that my negative self-thoughts began to shift. I did this by really questioning myself and those negative beliefs when they popped into my head. Internal conversations I had with myself might have gone something like this:

Negative Thought: *The new neighbor asked me if I was "just" a stay-at-home mom and when I said yes, I saw slight disdain flash within her eyes. I'm such a loser! I should have never quit my job.*

Positive Challenge: *Are you kidding me, Cook? With all the research out there that you've read, in addition your personal experience with children and what you know of cognitive development, you know the most important place for you right now is home full-time with the babies. Parenthood isn't a thankless job. Society thanks you every time they compliment you on how polite the kids are, how well they behave, and how happy and healthy they look. Being home is where you need to be right now and it won't be forever. In a few years when the kids start school, you can begin getting back into the workforce and reclaim your professional identity.*

Yes, these pep talks worked to rewire my brain and I don't have *as many* negative thoughts now. It took hundreds of these talks though... and I really had to start believing what I was saying.

What has worked even more than my own positive self-talk is when a stranger compliments me on my children's behavior. For instance, a receptionist at a doctor's office once said to me, "You stay home full-time, right? I can tell because your children look at people when they speak to them and have manners."

On other occasions, strangers on the street or in stores will spontaneously tell me what lovely children I have and how well they listen. These moments reinforce what the research says, which is being an actively involved parent with babies is very important, but it also lets me know that the amount of effort I put into providing the support they constantly need at this age is paying off.

I'm one of the lucky few in a profession where my value goes up merely by aging; most people like "seasoned" therapists. My educational background or experience didn't matter, when I looked younger. "What do you know about life? You're like, twelve," types of comments were occasionally thrown my way by a client.

Back to my point, whilst I felt a loss of identity, I didn't feel the pressure to hurry up and get back in the work game because I could use what I was learning during my time home with the babies to become a better psychologist (and write a book!).

Many professions aren't set-up for parents to easily take time away from work to be with their children and anticipate a smooth return back into the workforce. Yet more and more companies are beginning to read the research and offer in-house daycare, paid maternity *and* paternity leave, encouraging employees to take vacations and offer family events.

Even if you aren't the primary parent who stays home full-time, you will still go through changes in your identity. One of my cousins jokingly said he was gonna be a "weekend dad", that is until his awesome feminist wife wasn't having any of it and made him help with everything with their twin boys.

He hadn't been expecting to be going to work tired, losing the freedom to go play soccer on the weekends or head to the city for a boys' night out. He was committed to the weekend dad part but ended up being a full-time dad (which is what all dads should be anyway). Even though he was prepared for a new identity he ended up getting a different, more intense one, and he couldn't be happier, well... most of the time.

Whilst I thought I was prepared for the changes a baby would bring to life, I wasn't prepared for the deep and (sometimes) depressing realities that came with the loss of my identity. I was forced to face my own unrealistic expectations for myself, motherhood and parenthood. My self-esteem was negatively impacted by my negative views about stay-at-home parents. I had to challenge my distorted view of the value of the person who stays home and replace those thoughts with positive ones to rewire my brain.

It's really difficult to undo negative thoughts, but remember it is possible. Our brains are malleable which means we can create new neural pathways by merely shifting our perspective and by challenging old thoughts and ideas that don't make us feel good about ourselves. The concept is simple, but implementing it is sometimes difficult. I tell myself every day that I am doing the hardest, most important job out there and only recently have I started to believe it.

Chapter 26

BABY BLUES

It's Normal to Not Feel Normal

I WAS PROBABLY AROUND 15 years old when a story about a mother killing herself and her four children was being discussed during a female-only church activity. I don't remember exactly what we were doing, probably a service project of some sort, or learning how to be a "good wife and mother". Don't get me wrong, that last sentence wasn't sarcastic. I am grateful for my Mormon upbringing because one thing the Mormon Church does quite well is provide clear behavioral guidelines for how to raise children and help create successful families. Just take away the religious content and you can find loads of great ideas to do with babies/kids, as well as basic behavioral interventions and ideas to make your family system run smoothly.

Anyway, back to the "baby killer" that these ladies were discussing. They couldn't believe "…a woman in her right mind would kill her children." "Who does such a thing? Who? Tell me who?" Apparently, this poor soul was the mother of four kids ranging in age from 1-5 years old. She lived with her "very religious" and abusive husband off the grid in the country somewhere remote.

I'm guessing she probably felt this earthly world could offer no peace or love, and she had lost complete hope of a better life for herself and her children. So, instead of committing suicide and leaving her children to be abused and neglected by her husband, she takes them with her to a place where peace is promised to all who believe... or something like that.

Here's the thing. Being the primary parent of a tiny human requires sooooo much giving that individuals who don't have a support system, or who suffer from a mental/physical illness, or even those healthy "normal" functioning women, can experience bouts of feeling blue, postpartum depression, and even psychosis after a baby is born. It's exhausting watching a little human 24/7 and at the end (or beginning) of the day when all your resources and energy have been spent, sometimes it doesn't matter if you have someone to support you or not, you are an empty shell of a human.

I don't ever expect my kids to "appreciate all I do" for them (we've all heard our parents say that, right?). My children didn't ask me to be born so why take my frustrations out on them? I actually thought I had prepared myself for the selflessness that is required for parenting, but I had no clue.

When I was single and dating around, I used to tell everyone that when I was ready to be a little less selfish, I would consider marrying someone, and when I was ready to be completely selfless I would have kids. I was known as the baby whisperer at church from a young age and always thought I knew what I needed to know before having my own kids. Boy was I mistaken.

Being a psychologist, I had learned all about postpartum depression and its signs; I cognitively understood how the hormonal changes in a woman's body can make them emotional labile and create changes in sleep. I even thought I was ready for the full-time dependency this little person expected of me. Then my mother-in-law was unexpectedly given weeks to live.

Nothing trumps a dying parent, not even a newborn baby. My wife talked to her mother almost daily and was fortunate enough to work for a company that had an office in London so she could fly back and forth quite easily without missing work.

This meant that I was a single parent with Arthur for a cumulative total of 60 days whilst my partner attended to her dying mother. Arthur and I went over four times so he could know his Nana Jana and she could know him before she passed.

During this time, I never thought about harming Arthur. But my mind went to some very deep, dark existential places. My immediate family lived 2 hours away and my friends either had jobs or new babies, or jobs and new babies. If I'm honest, my pride also limited me from reaching out more. Remember, in my mind I should be able to "do it all" without support, or people would think I was weak. That's what cognitive behavioral psychologists call an "irrational thought", and it totally was.

Asking for help is NOT weak. I know this, and I've said it thousands of times to clients, friends, and family, even strangers for goodness' sake. Nevertheless, I struggle asking for help; I knew I had access to help and that knowledge in and of itself did provide a sense of peace. But I reflect on those single mothers, or parents who don't have anyone in their lives they feel close enough to, to lean on during the early years with children, and my heart and mind ache for them.

I can't imagine what life for me would have been like if I didn't have a safety net of friends and family. The Baby Blues are real and can happen to parents because no matter how much you prepare, until the baby arrives you just don't know how your life will change. Postpartum depression is real and every new parent (birth or adopted), is going through massive changes in their life. Those already prone toward depressive thoughts or anxiety experience those feelings even more after a baby arrives. Finally, postpartum *psychosis* is real and research states it happens in .1-.2% of women, but my hunch is it happens much more but is underreported because of the fear of "the system" taking a child away.

Those times my partner was out of the country for a week at a time, I would call my neighbors and invite Arthur and I over around 5:00 PM because it was at this point in the day that I just couldn't spend one more minute alone with the baby. I think most babies start to get fussy toward the end of their day, and I was over the 24/7 of having a baby without a break. I desperately needed a 30-minute break before starting the bed routine and so I reached out. Everyone happily had us over and it was wonderful.

I truly believe that unless you are the primary parent for a minimum of 2 months straight (with partner support if possible), you simply will not be able to grasp just how awful, lonely, difficult, strenuous and maddening being the primary parent can be.

Many primary parents talk about how their co-parent will watch the kid(s) for a day on the weekend (or even a whole weekend) and then talk about how much "fun" they had, how "easy" naps and put-downs were, and how it was pure bliss. (Puke, puke, puke.) Yes, maybe the stars aligned, and the co-parent had an easy time. It does happen once in a blue moon. But if you are the spouse reading this, please don't ever compare a short (even week long) period of time against what a primary parent of a baby/small child goes through day after day, month after month.

I'm sorry; until you live it you won't understand it. Validate the primary parent's experience whatever it is because at the end of the day we all experience things differently and it's just not nice, and it's counterproductive to argue over whom has it worse: the primary or co-parent.

New parents *need* support and to know they are not alone in their struggles. The woman I spoke about at the beginning of this chapter may have had postpartum psychosis/depression or even the Baby Blues. At the end of the day we will never know, but we do know she felt life on this Earth with her four children was worse than whatever fate she and her children would face as she drove herself and kids into a pond. Be kind to new parents, be nice, be supportive and be understanding. Babies/young toddlers are adorable but they sure are hard work.

Chapter 27

THE DUCHESS OF CAMBRIDGE DOES IT
Comparisons Will Kill the Parenting Vibe

IT'S CUSTOMARY TO WAIT until a person is 3 months pregnant before making the announcement to friends and family because the first 12 weeks of pregnancy have the highest occurrences of miscarriage. So, when I found out that the Duchess of Cambridge was pregnant and due 2 weeks before *my* little baby, the highly competitive, and often nonsensical, side of my brain kicked in.

Listen, sometimes we all have thoughts that we know aren't real (um... me competing with a duchess) and Cognitive Behavioral Theory (CBT) calls these thoughts cognitive distortions. These distortions can kick off a "negative loop of thinking" that often results in feeling badly about yourself.

CBT has identified several cognitive distortions most humans experience in some way or another... one of mine was what is called 'all or nothing' thinking. This means I see things that happen to me as either black or white, good or bad, as a success or a failure. An example of this is getting 80% on a test and saying you "failed" because you didn't get a perfect score. (Again, me in school. I would rather have gotten an "F" than a "B".)

My cognitive distortion was this: I was competing with the Duchess of Cambridge for who would have the healthiest, happiest, loveliest baby *first*. How did it make me feel? Stressed out and stupid for even thinking it. My partner and I would laugh about it because we both know how competitive I am and how silly this idea was.

Obviously, I didn't want to continue to have this absurd thought haunting me the rest of my life, so I knew I had to challenge it, face it, and try to understand why I was competing with her to begin with! She doesn't even know I exist, for goodness' sake.

One CBT technique for getting rid of cognitive distortions is what is called Socratic questioning. It's a specific way of asking questions which forces an individual to really challenge the validity of their irrational thought and come up with a "new" thought that is based in reality thereby alleviating the negative emotions caused by the irrational thought. Phew, did you get all that? In other words, forcing yourself to acknowledge the 80% you got on the test and admitting you didn't fail, but just didn't score as well as you wanted makes you feel better about the 20% loss.

Being married to a psychologist does have some benefits. My partner has picked up some 'psych' skills. So, when I started talking rubbish about competing with the Duchess of Cambridge, she immediately began challenging me on this thought and reminding me that the last time we had seen my mother she had mentioned the news about the royal baby but that 'her' grandbaby will be an even *better* prince than theirs.

My mother had brought up the competition without me even saying anything. This was the perfect place for my partner to continue the challenge/chat and at the very end of the chat, I realized that my "all or nothing" thinking all boiled down to this:

MY COGNITIVE DISTORTION

If I wasn't the best at everything, people would judge me as weak and therefore I would not be deserving of love.

What complete and utter nonsense, eh? Now I *know* and *believe* everyone in the world is deserving of love and respect, yet I didn't believe I was worthy of it unless I was perfect. My partner lovingly helped me realize, by talking it through, how silly I was being and how I was in fact VERY much loved by her and others. And she kindly reminded me that, "Nope, you're not perfect," but gave me a loving hug and said, "Neither am I."

This realization definitely helped me reframe and refocus my mindset about parenting before my children arrived, and it also helped me reflect on how my competitive side can often result in cognitive distortions that make me feel stressed/anxious and impact my entire life. I took a huge chill pill (metaphorically speaking) and tried hard to ignore all the comparison comments strangers made to me when I was in the UK with Arthur during the first year.

It was not easy because everyone, I'm talking *everyone,* seemed to have something to say to me about how much Arthur looked like the prince, or compared his age/size to the prince, and I would say, "Thank you," and try to just appreciate the compliment.

Oh, and just for the record, Arthur was born 2 weeks *before* Prince George and I *definitely* would have changed his name if it had matched because I could not cope with people asking if I had named him *after* the prince. We all have our limits, right?

I share this story with you because I'm not the first, nor will I be the last parent who feels like they are competing with other parents. If I had a dollar for every time a parent came into my office in tears because their child wasn't doing X, Y, Z like their peers, I would have most of my student loan paid off.

After carefully exploring the feelings these parents experienced, I realized they weren't upset that their child wasn't sitting on their own yet, but rather they were struggling to cope with their own feelings of inadequacy as a parent such as, "*I* must be doing something wrong at home because he is 3 weeks older than Z and *should* be sitting up."

When someone says something to you about your child and you feel an immediate emotional response, chances are you're reacting to one of your own issues... try to reflect on those incidents and examine them, and really question them. Read up on CBT techniques; get a CBT workbook for identifying cognitive distortions and start challenging them.

Did I completely stop thinking about the Duchess of Cambridge? Um, no, of course not. But when I started down one of my negative thought loops I would take a step back and recognize how silly I was being and tell my partner what the thought was, such as "... I was first to have a second baby~ whoot whoot!"

At parks, preschools, grocery stores, family events, and even on the sidewalk people are going to make comments about your child. Most of the time I believe people are just trying to make a connection with you and your little one when they say things like, "Oh, isn't your baby so adorable? How old are they? Oh really! Thirteen months! And they aren't walking yet? Oh, my grandson was walking at 10 months old. Don't worry, darling, they will walk when they are ready." Um, okay. I wasn't worried until you told me *not* to be worried random-stranger-who-gives-unsolicited-advice-for-free-on-the-street.

What *do* you do when someone says something that triggers you or that is an obvious slight or dig? I will explain it to you in a joke. The below is a conversation between two women from the deep south (so read it in your mind with a real reeeeal southern accent):

Lady 1- Congratulations on your first baby!

Lady 2- Thank you!

Lady 1- When I had my first baby, my husband bought me a new car.

Lady 2- How nice!

Lady 1- And when I had my second baby, he bought me a lake cottage!

Lady 2- How nice!

Lady 1- And when I had my *third* baby, he bought me a yacht!

Lady 2- How nice!

Lady 1- What did your husband buy you when you had your first baby?

Lady 2- Charm lessons.

Lady 1- Charm lessons? What did you want those for?

Lady 2- So when women like you told me stories like those, I could say "How nice!" instead of "bullshit".

No, you aren't going to respond to someone with "bullshit" when they say their child did X, but you *may* remember this joke and be able to, in your mind, smile and acknowledge that you don't need to compete with every person out there. Most of the time, you can just say things like:

Oh, that's nice.
Thank you for noticing.
Very good of you to say!

My goal for this chapter was to poke fun at myself and at the same time show you how to start learning about yourself from negative experiences with people regarding your kid(s).

At the end of the day, you really should only be competing with yourself... be more patient, kind and caring. We are so so *so* hard on ourselves and that translates into being a jerk to ourselves, and sometimes to others. Plus, these negative thoughts that arise when people start comparing young kids are stressful! Stop the stress by stopping the thoughts.

Try to focus on you and your baby, and your relationship with your partner and only let "others" into that tight little close-knit family if you want them or need them. Remember, most of the time people are trying to help. It just doesn't always feel that way. Smile, and remember to tell them... how nice... it was to see them again.

Chapter 28

DIVERSITY AND FAMILIES
Families Don't Look Like They Used to

SOMETIMES PEOPLE "OOPS" INTO parenthood while many others feel a social/biological calling to become parents. No matter how your child came to be, once they entered your life you became a family unit. What exactly defines a family? The Merriam-Webster dictionary defines family as:

The basic unit in society traditionally consisting of two parents rearing their children; also, any of various social units differing from but regarded as equivalent to the traditional family such as a single-parent family.

Families today look very different than the white, hetero couple with the 2.5 kids and a dog that Hollywood has displayed and held as the "American Ideal" for years. Please, don't get offended and all worked up and think I've got something against a "traditional" family, I don't! It's just that when other types of families (single parent, interracial couple, homosexual couple, foster parents, grandma and grandpa as primary parents, etc.) are successfully raising happy, healthy kids then these families need to be recognized and celebrated too. At the end of the day, it's discrimination and ignorance that harms children, not having two loving parents who may identify on the LGBTQ spectrum or those that were raised by a single parent and/or grandparent.

Listen, I once got into a heated debate with a friend from my childhood who is still *very* much a proud Mormon. He and I went back and forth and around the block again showing each other research papers which supported our opposing claims. (He believes, like some that children raised by same-sex parents suffer because of it. I don't.)

He and I finally agreed to "disagree", but our debate had sparked others on our social media accounts to chime in and that in and of itself made the debate worth it to me. Why? Because people (from all walks of life) stopped and took notice that these two *very* different people could have a polite, considerate, respectful discussion about a very touchy topic: gay parenting.

When it's all said and done, I strongly believe that two people, who love each other, respect each other and cherish their children, can never go wrong. Two people, who disrespect each other, are in a cycle of abuse, and/or fight all the time should *not* be modeling that type of behavior for their child.

Get a divorce, separate or whatever, and allow the distance between the two of you to clear the air enough so you can get yourself together and model how to be respectful of another human being to your child. Research states kids are better off when parents in a toxic relationship separate. Just saying.

Back to diversity and families. Children learn what we teach them. If we teach and *model* tolerance and acceptance, then that is what our children learn. If we teach and *model* discrimination and hate, then that is what our children learn. To really be accepting of diversity in families, one has to reflect on what it is that you believe constitutes a family. Does it *have* to be a man and a woman, or could it be something else? How is your family similar/different from other families?

When my partner and I hooked up and before things got really serious, we talked about our feelings about having kids and becoming parents. She quickly responded to me that since she had come out as a lesbian, she had stopped thinking about having kids because she thought it would be too hard on the child, due to *SOCIETY'S* pressures. She knew that two loving people could care for and raise amazing humans, but she feared for how "the others" would see our children and tease them for having two moms.

I told her that children are teased every day about their eyes, nose, ears, teeth, if they smell, if they have freckles, if they are too fat or too thin, and yes, if their parents are gay. Our job as parents is to not shield our children from this type of abuse because we as humans all endure discrimination on some level or other from our peers as we grow and even as adults.

Instead of teaching our children to seek out "sameness" give them the confidence, language, and coping skills needed to help navigate the world of relationships with people and society that are different from them. Being different is good and the world needs variety... it's the spice of life! If only the best songbirds sang, our forests would be very quiet.

I've spent most of my life fighting to be my truest self, which meant I swam in the opposite direction of the mainstream. This type of swimming didn't build my muscles, but it did give me thick skin to endure insults slung at me and the endurance, perspective and vision to be able to pull back from a situation and really try to understand another person's experience of life.

Just doing that, putting yourself in another person's shoes, is what you need to do when you become a parent, not only for your child's sake, but so you can become more empathetic toward other parents and their families.

I promise you our similarities far outweigh the differences. Be real. Be accepting. Be understanding. Be open to all the colors and combinations of families today and embrace the love. Hate never wins; it only gives you indigestion and ulcers. Love always wins and it gives you happiness and joy. Choose wisely.

Chapter 29

PRIVILEGE AND PARENTING
It's Much More than You Think

I GREW UP SWIMMING in lakes, ponds, rivers, and creeks. You name it, I swam it. What I learned from those many experiences is the following: if you want to actually go for a swim in ice cold water (Lake Michigan runs around 58/60 degrees when I start swimming in the summer), the quicker you dive in, the easier it is to acclimate. Yes, your body is "shocked" and your brain tells you this might not be the best idea, but you persevere.

Then, once you've paddled around for a few minutes your body begins warming up and you think, "Hey, this water isn't *that* cold, I'm actually enjoying myself." And with the knowledge that you're getting exercise PLUS burning extra calories due to cold water, it makes that initial plunge into the water worth it, at least for me.

When I started waking up to the idea that people in this country and the world *aren't* treated the same simply because of the color of their skin or gender, I was initially very resistant to that idea. I actually laughed at a girlfriend of mine in 2002 when she told me she was pulled over because she was black. I've grown a LOT since then.

After my initial resistance (dipping my toe in the freezing water), I realized when it comes to waking up to the injustices of the world and how my silence merely continues to hurt others, I had to dive headfirst into the freezing cold water of looking at myself and my privilege and what it means to me and how I can use my platform of privilege to help others.

The term "just the tip of the iceberg" means you may notice something above the water, but the size of what you see is nothing compared to what lies beneath the icy waters. When speaking to the topic of privilege it's not difficult for us to see our own "tip of the iceberg" in ourselves when it comes to our privileges such as skin color, wealth, education, etc. Obviously, we can choose to look away from the mirror, or we can choose to look at it, change if needed, and hopefully better ourselves and those around us by acknowledging our privileges and using them to help others.

To see the *really, really* cold, frozen, often never explored area of your iceberg, you are gonna have to take a plunge, my friends into the icy water of self-exploration. It's a very scary place to go, I know. Soooo… tag, I'm it. I will go first, but before I do, I want to define the word *privilege*. You should know there are many dictionary definitions of privilege, but all have the same overall gist. This is the definition I am using:

> *privilege*: a special right, advantage, or immunity granted or available only to a particular person or group of people.

Now, I'm not going to go into details about every "ah-ha" moment I've had since my plunge and "wake up", but I will share a few moments in history about myself that I feel are relevant to parenting and privileges.

Referring back to the above definition of privilege, I want you to take note of the word *advantage*. Often when speaking on the topic of privilege words like gender, sex, and money get talked about a lot and they *should*. I will get back to those privileges and parenting later in this chapter, but first I want to point out a privilege you may not automatically consider about parenting which is this: how much exposure/opportunity have you had being around babies/young children *before* you became a parent? Unless you were born into a large family or a member of a group/community which encourages procreation and discourages contraception, your exposure to babies has more than likely been limited.

Remember in the very first chapter of this book where I mentioned I was raised Mormon in the Midwest? Let's go back there for a minute. Mormons are encouraged to have lots of babies *and* Mormons hang out at church functions at *least* twice a week, often for a minimum of 2 hours. So, from the age of 6 years old (when my parents joined), I was around babies and role models for dealing with and managing lots and lots of babies.

I had my first child at the age of 37 years old and had acquired by that time the following:

- 31 years of "hands on" experience with babies/kids/families
- a rough *minimum* of 9, 672 hours of hands-on experience/practice with babies/kids
- 16 years of higher education and internships geared toward learning about human behavior/families

The one thing I wish to make abundantly clear is this: *EVEN* with the above resume of exposure and knowledge about babies, my daily struggle to mentally survive was real. It was a *privilege* that I was adopted into a family who joined a community that offered so much exposure to babies/kids and techniques for managing them. It gave me the confidence and knowledge to feel ready to deal with my own children.

Many parents have had little to no exposure with babies before their own come, and therefore by default, are much more cautious with things like how to pick-up/hold their child, pat them hard enough to force out that stubborn burp, but not too hard to hurt them, how to change a diaper, how to breastfeed and so many other things.

I remember visiting my BFF and her first-born. She did not have a lot of exposure with babies growing up. So, after her baby was born, I went to visit to show her some of my baby "tricks". One thing she realized immediately was how comfortable I was handling a baby:

picking him up, moving him around (floppy head and all) and all the different carrying positions I knew (again thank the Mormon Church and all those babies and role models I grew up with). She even took a picture of me with her son slung across one arm like a sack of potatoes happily chilling in this "different" position whilst I held a glass of wine with the other hand.

She cried later in the day when he fell asleep on my chest as we sat and chatted because he had never done that with her before and watching how "easy" I made it look made her feel like a complete failure as a parent.

I lovingly reminded her that she literally had minimal experience holding babies and it was all brand new to her. She got better over time and was much more comfortable with baby #2. An important thing to remember is this: a baby can sense whether or not the person holding them is anxious or uncomfortable or if they are relaxed and calm. Because I've had the privilege of being around and holding babies most of my life I am *very* secure in my abilities and believe a baby can immediately sense that… they think, "Oooo, this bitch knows what's up so I'm gonna chill in her competent arms," or something like that.

No matter who you are (me included), your first-born child helps you work out/learn/practice/test all the "kinks" and if a second child comes, parents (me included), usually find it a little bit easier in general. Remember though, each child is very different because, well, they are their own unique person, so whilst you're more confident washing an infant (first-born in a special tub in the kitchen sink, subsequent babies shower in the arms of parents), you may not have as much experience with something else, such as coping with a baby who gets eight teeth at 6 months old.

Bottom line: your exposure (or lack thereof) to babies, role models, and practice time directly impacts where you begin on the invisible line of parenting. Some (like me), start out with a 50-yard *advantage* toward the arbitrary "end zone" of parenting because I've had the *privilege* of being raised in a community that exposed me to positive (for the most part), role models and hands-on experience being around young children and babies.

Okay, onto the next privilege I want to talk about which is a more obvious one, my skin color. In the drab, cold, grey days of winter in the city of Chicago my skin color is usually quite white, but still has a little color to it. In the summer, when I've been working outside a lot, I often can be mistaken for being of mixed race which I've always heard as a compliment, but that's a *privilege* in and of itself.

I am able to *"choose"* which racial group I want to belong to... meaning I could stop going in the sun and look "white" again or get a tan and be seen as mixed/exotic in my racial background (BTW I've done the genetic make-up test and I am almost 99% Eastern European). People of color never have the opportunity to hide their skin tone.

Why does the color of my skin matter, you ask? The color of my skin affords me privileges when it comes to, well, everything. Being a member of the most powerful racial group the developed world has ever known is a pretty big deal and a ton of free stuff comes with this privilege... I'm talking the ultimate "goodie-bag-from-an-Oscar-party" good.

The first person to be recorded as acknowledging privilege in this country was W.E.B. Du Bois (an African American) when he penned an essay talking about how African Americans were conscious of racial discrimination, but Caucasians were not aware because the systems (government, education, police, etc.), supported Caucasian culture/power.

Peggy McIntosh was teaching at Wellesley College in the 1980s and was the first person to categorize ways her skin color gave her an advantage in life. Since then many other types of privilege "checklists" have been created. Keep in mind that privilege isn't just about skin color but there are other elements to consider here like educational background, social class standing, and gender. Examining how *all* these marginalized groups overlap one another is called *intersectionality*.

Intersectionality is a term coined by another woman named Kimberle Crenshaw, who shows how privilege isn't just about one thing (race, gender, social status), but rather it involves the mixing/blending/overlapping of all of your social identities and how these identities either work in your favor or discriminate against you (institutions/governments).

You can be uneducated, male, poor and Caucasian. You can be educated, female, middle-class and black. These two people will *both* face discrimination, but the woman's life could arguably be more difficult *even though* she has an education and is middle-class *because* she is 1. female (difficult to hide gender) and 2. she is black (difficult to hide skin color). Both factors place her in marginalized groups of society.

At the end of the day you *will* have unearned advantages and unearned disadvantages simply due to a combination of factors that overlap and create your unique set of circumstances as an individual. It's your choice to either address these things or not, and I will say this from personal experience... it is not easy, but it is worth it.

I've pulled a few items off a list of privileges from Peggy McIntosh's original list and I want to write my experiences beside them to give you an example.

Some of my privileges (aside from those I've already mentioned):

1. I can readily find accurate (or non-caricatured) examples of members of my class depicted in films, books, television, and other media. *Most of the parenting books I've read are by educated Caucasian people, and I'm another one. Most of the shows my children watch, especially the "classics" like Mary Poppins, all depict a variety of characters that my children can identify with.*

2. I do not have to educate my children to be aware of systemic racism for their own daily physical protection. *YES, TRUE. Turn on the news and/or watch videos posted online. You will see children of color being handcuffed, harassed, killed even and treated inappropriately in other ways. I have already started talking to my children about how the color of their skin,*

hair, and eyes will give them advantages in life others don't have, and as they grow, I will teach them how to use this privilege to help others.

3. I can be pretty sure that my children's teachers and employers will tolerate them if they fit into school and workplace norms. My chief worries about them do not concern others' attitudes toward their race. *Yup.*

4. I can easily buy posters, postcards, picture books, greeting cards, dolls, toys and children's magazines featuring people of my race. *Again, very true. I have to actively seek out books about children from different ethnicities and cultures, so I can talk to my children about the importance of embracing diversity.*

5. I can worry about racism without being seen as self-interested or self-seeking. *How about a huge fat YES!*

6. I can be pretty sure of finding people who would be willing to talk with me and advise me about my next steps, professionally. *Another yes.*

7. I have no difficulty finding neighborhoods where people approve of our household. *IF I lived in the suburbs or a small town, my family might run into problems. As it is, we live in the diverse city of Chicago on a block with wonderful neighbors who love and accept our family.*

8. I will feel welcomed and "normal" in the usual walks of public life, institutional and social. *I absolutely do feel this way. Some might argue it's my gregarious personality that affords me the "extras" I get in life. Even if that WAS the case, I know I wouldn't feel as welcomed if I was a different color.*

As I mentioned earlier, these are just a sample of some of the things my privileges afford me. A few others include my educational background (I get instant respect from other professionals that work/interact with my children), access to affordable healthcare (my partner's company offers *amazing* healthcare, so I never have to make the awful choice of 1. taking my child to see a doctor/specialist or 2.

paying the electric bill) and my partner makes enough money so I *can* have the *choice* to stay home full-time with the children (we do have to budget to make it happen, but it's worth it for the first few years. I plan on going back to work once the youngest starts school full-time).

I've given you a few samples of the privileges I have just by being born Caucasian along with a few less obvious ones. At the end of the day, talking about these topics is not easy and looking at our own advantages and how they have helped us can provoke feelings of guilt, anger, frustration and sadness. That's completely normal and to be expected. As the saying goes, no pain no gain.

As you begin to "wake-up", those around you may become resistant to your changes because it will force them to also begin examining their lives and that can cause a chasm between you, or hopefully a bridge instead.

Personally, some of my relationships have been strained with friends and family because I can no longer be silent about my privileges and the suffering of others. *Especially* when simple things *could* be done to make life better for so many people, but the systems of suppression continue and those few at the top in power want to make sure those assuming power keep the status quo.

The only way the machine/system can change is if those at the controls change it. As I've said before, I am pretty high up on the pecking order and want to use my platform to highlight the need for self-awareness for other parents. It's not just about the color of your skin. Knowing your advantages and disadvantages in life is important because it impacts your parenting and how you raise your children.

It is not easy. I've learned that I carry a LOT of baggage from my past, and nine out of ten times my initial thought about people in situations where I feel threatened are often those nasty negative stereotypes I've seen/heard/experienced most of my life.

Good news is that the more "woke" I become the less angry and more understanding about others and their own plight I get. When it comes to parenting, I have a HUGE amount of empathy to parents of color, single parents, interracial parents and LGBTQ parents because these groups of parents will come up against barriers every day that other families won't.

I've been very blessed in my life and have always believed to whom much is given much is expected. As parents, we need to be aware of our advantages and seek ways to help each other in this game called parenthood.

Chapter 30

FOR WHAT IT'S WORTH
It's Worth It

AS YOU KNOW BY now, I always wanted kids. I will never really know what came first, my desire or society telling me to want babies. Regardless, I have two special little humans and now that I am getting regular sleep I feel like I'm outta the woods (both kids older than 24 months). My life did not turn out like I thought it would, but I sure am glad it turned out the way it did.

I have been writing short notes and recording thoughts since Arthur was a baby about my experiences during the first few years with my children. My experiences are not uncommon, but I didn't find many people talk about the more mundane and stressful parts of being with a young human 24/7. They would just say, "Oh, it goes by in the blink of an eye." Yeah, maybe it does, but when you are exhausted, hungry, have needed to use the loo for the past 45 minutes and your infant has just exploded shit everywhere in the middle of a diaper change, time goes *very, very slooooooooowly.*

Consequently, the very second I realized I felt human again I knew I had to get this book written or I would start to forget just how awful… painfully awful… it was at times with a child from 0-2 years old. This book was my therapy and kept me sane while the kids were younger. Not only was I able to say to people, "Yes, I stay home full-time and

I'm writing a book about parenting," but it also gave my brain something else to focus on while waiting for my kid to slowly climb the stairs.

I seriously was shocked at just how hard I found my first few years at home with the kids… granted I had two 19 months apart. It *completely* blew until Ivy was around 2, but now the kids are thick as thieves. I believe parents play a huge role in helping their children learn how to build, maintain and flourish in sibling relationships, and I will talk more about this in my next book which will look at the ages of 3-5.

My children are older now and able to do things when I tell them to, like, "Go wash your hands before lunch," rather than me needing to move them around in a baby bouncer whilst I picked the weeds in the garden.

I really do love being a parent, but that title is not the whole of me but rather a part of me. All the crap we go through as parents is just unreal. Nevertheless, I believe it is worth it. Your journey will be different than mine, but just as real and just as unique as you and your family. I believe the sacrifice I am making to prepare two more humans to face life as prepared as they can be (mentally, physically, emotionally and spiritually), is valuable. It is worth it to me because I know I matter to my children and they make me want to be a better person.

This book is my contribution to the fight for love and understanding trumping hate and violence. The ultimate goal is to provide ways to become better parents who in turn will raise stronger, more resilient children that grow-up and foster a kinder, more tolerant world. This monumental change starts by planting one tiny little seed in the mind of a new parent and if this book shifts your perspective on one (or many) things about parenting for the better, then indeed great things can happen but it starts at home…

ACKNOWLEDGEMENTS

FIRST AND FOREMOST THIS book would not have been possible without the constant loving and caring support of my partner, Zoe. You have been a solid rock and a provider throughout not only the writing of this book but also my entire doctorate educational training *and* after the arrival of the babies. You continue to support all of my "crazy" ideas and dreams by remaining strong in your commitment to our children and me. My life changed for the better the moment I met you and I couldn't ask for a better partner in this game called life. Thank you.

Dearest children, even though you are still too young to comprehend what I am writing, someday you will be old enough to read and understand this book. I want to tell you that none of this would have been possible without you. You have taught me what it means to love unconditionally and you've tolerated my growing pains as I added the job title "parent" to my resume. As with any new job there are always kinks that need to be worked out. You both have happily forgiven me my shortcomings and helped me grow into a better person. For this I can never repay you. Thank you.

I must acknowledge and thank my parents. I know I was not an easy child to raise with my energy and sassy mouth. Dad, you've always been there for me and supported and encouraged me in all of my life choices, thank you. Mom, thank you for teaching me how to be resilient and strong in the face of adversity, for modeling how to *not give a damn* what other people think and to not be afraid of hearing the word *no*.

Rachel, I don't even know where to start with you. Within minutes of meeting you for the first time and after learning that you were an English major/editor, I asked you to edit this book, which at the time was merely 2 chapters. Without hesitation you said *yes*. Not only have you been an amazing editor but you've morphed into a dear friend that I can't live without. You were always there with a kind word or inspirational text when I was feeling low and frustrated with the writing process. The suggestions you made were always given kindly and with thoughtful purpose. You encouraged me to be true to my "own voice" in how I wrote and brilliantly made my dyslexic writing style flow seamlessly. Where would I be without you and your guidance! Thank you.

Of course, I must thank my friend Sharon for reading the entire book twice! Your fresh set of eyes were able to see things that might have gone unnoticed. You've helped me tighten up the book even more and I appreciate your feedback and willingness to help.

It's been an amazing, adventurous, exciting roller coaster of a relationship with you my BFF, Katie. Little did I know the lasting and profound impact you would have on my life when we met at the young age of 18. Throughout all the "growing pains" of becoming an adult we had each other to lean on. There is no doubt in my mind that I would not be the person I am today if we hadn't met so many years ago. Thank you so very much for your steady and unwavering support.

Where would I be without you Robin? I don't know how I would have mentally survived had you not been so gracious and selfless with your time and love during the early years with the children. Your husband Stan has also been a lifesaver for my family on so many occasions. Stan, you are a man of action and intellect which means you can always "fix the unfixable". Knowing that you both are just across the street or a phone call away provides more peace of mind than you will ever know. Thank you.

Last but definitely not least (and in no particular order), I want to thank my extended family, friends, professors/teachers, clients and acquaintances. Being the type of person who thrives from being real and true with people is the only way I know how to exist. I've felt continued support throughout my life and all of you have somehow imprinted yourself into my understanding and appreciation for life and family. Many of you have voluntarily bared your soul to me, and I thank you for your bravery. To those of you who have been strong enough for me to feel safe with you and show weakness, fragility, powerlessness and helplessness, I am forever in your debt. Thank you.

For What It's Worth
Bibliography

Abate, M. (2008). *Tomboys: A Literary and Cultural History*. Temple University Press.

Adair, L., Popkin, B., & Guilkey, D. (1993). The Duration of Breast-Feeding: How Is It Affected by Biological, Sociodemographic, Health Sector, and Food Industry Factors? *Demography, 30*(1), 63-80.

American College of Obstetricians and Gynecologists. Labor and delivery. (2015). In: Your Pregnancy and Childbirth Month to Month. 6th ed. Washington, D.C.: American College of Obstetricians and Gynecologists.

Amsalem, D., Hasson-Ohayon, I., Gothelf, D., & Roe, D. (2018). Subtle ways of stigmatization among professionals: The subjective experience of consumers and their family members. *Psychiatric Rehabilitation Journal, 41(3)*, 163-168.

Aneshensel, C., Frerichs, R., & Clark, V. (1981). Family Roles and Sex Differences in Depression. *Journal of Health and Social Behavior, 22* (4), 379-393.

Armstrong, T. (1977). The Brain: Its Relationship to Learning, Emotional States, and Behavior. *The American Biology Teacher,39* (4), 224-226.

Aunola, K., & Nurmi, J. (2005). The Role of Parenting Styles in Children's Problem Behavior. *Child Development, 76*(6), 1144-1159.

Barnhill, A., & Morain, S. (2015). Latch On or Back Off? Public Health, Choice, and the Ethics of Breast-Feeding Promotion Campaigns. *International Journal of Feminist Approaches to Bioethics, 8*(2), 139-171.

Baumrind, D. (1966). Effects of Authoritative Parental Control on Child Behavior. *Child Development, 37*(4), 887-907.

Baumrind, D., & Black, A. (1967). Socialization Practices Associated with Dimensions of Competence in Preschool Boys and Girls. *Child Development, 38*(2), 291-327.

Baumrind, D. (1997). Necessary Distinctions. *Psychological Inquiry, 8*(3), 176-182.

Beck, J. (2011). *Cognitive Behavior Therapy, Second Edition: Basics and Beyond: 2nd edition.* New York: Guilford Press.

Beckman, L., & Houser, B. (1979). Perceived Satisfactions and Costs of Motherhood and Employment among Married Women. *Journal of Population, 2*(4), 306-327.

Bell, S., & Ainsworth M. (1972). Infant Crying and Maternal Responsiveness. *Child Development, 43*(4), 1171-1190.

Belsky, J., Hancox, R. J., Sligo, J., & Poulton, R. (2012). Does being an older parent attenuate the intergenerational transmission of parenting? *Developmental Psychology, 48*(6), 1570-1574.

Bentley, A. (2006). Booming Baby Food: Infant Food and Feeding in Post-World War II America. *Michigan Historical Review, 32*(2), 63-87.

Berger, M. (1979). Men's New Family Roles: Some Implications for Therapists. *The Family Coordinator, 28*(4), 638-646.

Bernier, A., Carlson, S., Bordeleau, S., & Carrier, J. (2010). Relations Between Physiological and Cognitive Regulatory Systems: Infant Sleep Regulation and Subsequent Executive Functioning. *Child Development, 81*(6), 1739-1752.

Berger, L. (2007). Socioeconomic Factors and Substandard Parenting. *Social Service Review, 81*(3), 485-522.

Bernstein, R. E., Laurent, H. K., Measelle, J. R., Hailey, B. C., & Ablow, J. C. (2013). Little tyrants or just plain tired: Evaluating attributions for caregiving outcomes across the transition to parenthood. *Journal of Family Psychology, 27*(6), 851-861.

Best, J., & Miller, P. (2010). A Developmental Perspective on Executive Function. *Child Development, 81*(6), 1641-1660.

Biehle, S. N., & Mickelson, K. D. (2012). First-time parents' expectations about the division of childcare and play. *Journal of Family Psychology, 26*(1), 36-45.

Bisping, R., Steingrueber, H., Oltmann, M., & Wenk, C. (1990). Adults' Tolerance of Cries: An Experimental Investigation of Acoustic Features. *Child Development, 61*(4), 1218-1229.

Blumberg, M. S., Gall, A. J., & Todd, W. D. (2014). The development of sleep–wake rhythms and the search for elemental circuits in the infant brain. *Behavioral Neuroscience, 128*(3), 250-263.

Bocknek, E. L., Richardson, P. A., van den Heuvel, M. I., Qipo, T., & Brophy-Herb, H. E. (2018). Sleep moderates the association between routines and emotion regulation for toddlers in poverty. *Journal of Family Psychology, 32*(7), 966-974.

Boergers, J., Hart, C., Owens, J. A., Streisand, R., & Spirito, A. (2007). Child sleep disorders: Associations with parental sleep duration and daytime sleepiness. *Journal of Family Psychology, 21*(1), 88-94.

Bornstein, M., Putnick, D., Joan T. D. Suwalsky, & Gini, M. (2006). Maternal Chronological Age, Prenatal and Perinatal History, Social Support, and Parenting of Infants. *Child Development, 77*(4), 875-892.

Botto, S. V., & Rochat, P. (2018). Sensitivity to the evaluation of others emerges by 24 months. *Developmental Psychology, 54*(9), 1723-1734.

Bowen, M. (1985). *Family Therapy in Clinical Practice.* Lanham, Maryland: Roman and Littlefield Publisher.

Boyd, R., & Silk, J.B., (2000). *How Humans Evolved* (2nd edn). New York: W.W. Norton and Company.

Bradley, R., McKelvey, L., & Whiteside-Mansell, L. (2011). Does the Quality of Stimulation and Support in the Home Environment Moderate the Effect of Early Education Programs? *Child Development, 82*(6), 2110-2122.

Brenning, K., Soenens, B., & Vansteenkiste, M. (2015). What's your motivation to be pregnant? Relations between motives for parenthood and women's prenatal functioning. *Journal of Family Psychology, 29*(5), 755-765.

Broman, C. (1991). Gender, Work-Family Roles, and Psychological Well-Being of Blacks. *Journal of Marriage and Family, 53*(2), 509-520.

Brooks, R., & Obrzut, J. (1981). Brain Lateralization: Implications for Infant Stimulation and Development. *Young Children, 36*(3), 9-16.

Brown, S. (2017). *Families in America*. Oakland, California: University of California Press.

Buckhalt, J., El-Sheikh, M., & Keller P. (2007). Children's Sleep and Cognitive Functioning: Race and Socioeconomic Status as Moderators of Effects. *Child Development, 78*(1), 213-231.

Budnick, C. J., & Barber, L. K. (2015). Behind sleepy eyes: Implications of sleep loss for organizations and employees. *Translational Issues in Psychological Science, 1*(1), 89-96.

Burleson, B. R., Denton, W. H., (1992). A new look at similarity and attraction in marriage: Similarities in social-cognitive and communication skills as predictors of attraction and satisfaction. *Communication Monographs, 59*, 268–287.

Brooks C., Bolzendahl C., (2004). The transformation of US gender role attitudes: Cohort replacement, social-structural change, and ideological learning. *Social Science Research,33,* 106–133

Byars, K. C., & Simon, S. L. (2016). Behavioral treatment of pediatric sleep disturbance: Ethical considerations for pediatric psychology practice. *Clinical Practice in Pediatric Psychology, 4*(2), 241-248.

C. F. Zachariah Boukydis, & Burgess, R. (1982). Adult Physiological Response to Infant Cries: Effects of Temperament of Infant, Parental Status, and Gender. *Child Development, 53*(5), 1291-1298.

Cahill, S. (2009). The Disproportionate Impact of Antigay Family Policies on Black and Latino Same-sex Couple Households. *Journal of African American Studies, 13*(3), 219-250.

Campos, B., Wang, S., Plaksina, T., Repetti, R. L., Schoebi, D., Ochs, E., & Beck, M. E. (2013). Positive and negative emotion in the daily life of dual-earner couples with children. *Journal of Family Psychology, 27*(1), 76-85.

Cao, H., Zhou, N., Leerkes, E. M., & Qu, J. (2018). Multiple domains of new mothers' adaptation: Interrelations and roots in childhood maternal non-supportive emotion socialization. *Journal of Family Psychology, 32*(5), 575-587.

Caporael, L., Dawes, R. M., Orbell, J. M., and van de Kragt, A. J. C., (1989). Selfishness examined: cooperation in the absence of egoistic incentives. *Behavioral and Brain Sciences, 12,* 683-739.

Cardenas, R., & Major, D. (2005). Combining Employment and Breastfeeding: Utilizing a Work-Family Conflict Framework to Understand Obstacles and Solutions. *Journal of Business and Psychology, 20*(1), 31-51.

Casey, S. J., Solomons, L. C., Steier, J., Kabra, N., Burnside, A., Pengo, M. F. Kopelman, M. D. (2016). Slow wave and REM sleep deprivation effects on explicit and implicit memory during sleep. *Neuropsychology, 30*(8), 931-945.

Carlson, M., & Corcoran, M. (2001). Family Structure and Children's Behavioral and Cognitive Outcomes. *Journal of Marriage and Family, 63*(3), 779-792.

Carr, C. (1998). Tomboy Resistance and Conformity: Agency in Social Psychological Gender Theory. *Gender and Society, 12*(5), 528-553.

Clark, C. A., & Smith, P. R. (2009). Promoting collaborative practice for children of parents with mental illness and their families. *Psychiatric Rehabilitation Journal, 33*(2), 95-97.

Clark, D. A., Klump, K. L., & Burt, S. A. (2018). Parent depressive symptomatology moderates the etiology of externalizing behavior in childhood: An examination of gene-environment interaction effects. *Developmental Psychology, 54*(7), 1277-1289.

Clarke-Stewart, K. (1973). Interactions between Mothers and Their Young Children: Characteristics and Consequences. *Monographs of the Society for Research in Child Development,38*(6/7), 1-109.

Chapman, G. (1992) *The 5 Love Languages: The Secret to Love that Lasts.* Chicago, Illinois: Northfield Publishing.

CHEVALIER, J. (2002). Frontal Lobes, Limbic Processing, Implicit Learning. In *Corpus and the Cortex: The 3-D Mind, Volume 2* (pp. 29-42). McGill-Queen's University Press.

Collins, C., Ryan, P., Crowther, C., McPhee, A., Paterson, S., & Hiller, J. (2004). Effect Of Bottles, Cups, And Dummies On Breast Feeding In Preterm Infants: Randomised Controlled Trial. *BMJ: British Medical Journal, 329*(7459), 193-196.

Connelly, J., Appleby, L., Robinson, J., Beech, B., & Griffith, P. (1991). Suicide During And After Pregnancy [with Reply]. *BMJ: British Medical Journal, 302*(6776), 591-592.

Cooklin, A. R., Giallo, R., D'Esposito, F., Crawford, S., & Nicholson, J. M. (2013). Postpartum maternal separation anxiety, overprotective parenting, and children's social-emotional well-being: Longitudinal evidence from an Australian cohort. *Journal of Family Psychology, 27*(4), 618-628.

Crenshaw, K. (1989) Demarginalizing the Intersection of Race and Sex: A Black Feminist Critique of Antidiscrimination Doctrine, Feminist Theory and Antiracist Politics. *University of Chicago Legal Forum: 1,* 8.

Crockenberg, S. (1981). Infant Irritability, Mother Responsiveness, and Social Support Influences on the Security of Infant-Mother Attachment. *Child Development, 52*(3), 857-865.

Croizet, J.-C., Després, G., Gauzins, M.-E., Huguet, P., Leyens, J.-P., & Méot, A. (2004). Stereotype Threat Undermines Intellectual Performance by Triggering a Disruptive Mental Load. *Personality and Social Psychology Bulletin, 30*(6), 721–731.

Crosnoe, R., Wirth, R., Pianta, R., Leventhal, T., Pierce, K., & NICHD Early Child Care. (2010). Family Socioeconomic Status and Consistent Environmental Stimulation in Early Childhood. *Child Development, 81*(3), 972-987.

Cutas, D. (2011). On triparenting. Is having three committed parents better than having only two? *Journal of Medical Ethics,37*(12), 735-738.

D'Souza, J., & Gurin, M. (2016). The universal significance of Maslow's concept of self-actualization. *The Humanistic Psychologist, 44*(2), 210-214.

De Jong, M., Verhoeven, M., Hooge, I. T. C., Maingay-Visser, A. P. G. F., Spanjerberg, L., & van Baar, A. L. (2018). Cognitive functioning in toddlerhood: The role of gestational age, attention capacities, and maternal stimulation. *Developmental Psychology, 54*(4), 648-662.

Darwin, C. (1871). *The decent of man, and selection in relation to sex* (2 vols). London: John Murray.

Daugherty, L., Dossani, R., Johnson, E., & Wright, C. (2014). Moving Beyond Screen Time: Redefining Developmentally Appropriate Technology Use in Early Childhood Education. In *Moving Beyond Screen Time:*

Redefining Developmentally Appropriate Technology Use in Early Childhood Education (pp. 1-8). RAND Corporation.

Davis, M. (2007). Neural Systems Involved in Fear and Anxiety Based on the Fear-potentiated startle test. *Neurobiology of Learning and Memory,* 381-425.

Davidov, M., & Grusec, J. (2006). Untangling the Links of Parental Responsiveness to Distress and Warmth to Child Outcomes. *Child Development, 77*(1), 44-58.

DAVIDSON, M. (2015). Experts in Birth: How Doulas Improve Outcomes for Birthing Women and Their Babies. In DAVIS-FLOYD R. (Author) & Castañeda A. & Searcy J. (Eds.), *Doulas and Intimate Labour: Boundaries, Bodies, and Birth* (pp. 15-31). BRADFORD, ONTARIO: Demeter Press.

Deater-Deckard, K. (2004). Parenting Behavior and the Parent-Child Relationship. In *Parenting Stress* (pp. 74-94). NEW HAVEN; LONDON: Yale University Press.

Deater-Deckard, K. (2004). *Parenting Stress.* NEW HAVEN; LONDON: Yale University Press.

Denissen, J. J. A., Luhmann, M., Chung, J. M., & Bleidorn, W. (2018). Transactions between life events and personality traits across the adult lifespan. *Journal of Personality and Social Psychology.* Advance online publication.

Diamond, Adele. (2012). Activities and programs that improve children's executive functions. *Current Directions in Psychological Science, 21*(5): 335-41.

Diamond, D. J., & Diamond, M. O. (2017). Parenthood after reproductive loss: How psychotherapy can help with postpartum adjustment and parent–infant attachment. *Psychotherapy, 54*(4), 373-379.

Dictionary.com Unabridged Based on the Random House Unabridged Dictionary, © Random House, Inc. 2018

Dishion, T., Connell, A., Weaver, C., Shaw, D., Gardner, F., & Wilson, M. (2008). The Family Check-Up with High-Risk Indigent Families: Preventing Problem Behavior by Increasing Parents' Positive Behavior Support in Early Childhood. *Child Development, 79*(5), 1395-1414.

Dolbin-MacNab, M. (2006). Just Like Raising Your Own? Grandmothers' Perceptions of Parenting a Second Time Around. *Family Relations, 55*(5), 564-575.

Don, B. P., & Mickelson, K. D. (2012). Paternal postpartum depression: The role of maternal postpartum depression, spousal support, and relationship satisfaction. *Couple and Family Psychology: Research and Practice, 1*(4), 323-334.

Donovan, W., & Leavitt, L. (1989). Maternal Self-Efficacy and Infant Attachment: Integrating Physiology, Perceptions, and Behavior. *Child Development, 60*(2), 460-472.

Dowling, S., Pontin, D., & Boyer, K. (Eds.). (2018). *Social experiences of breastfeeding: Building bridges between research, policy and practice.* Bristol, UK; Chicago, IL, USA: Bristol University Press.

Dunbar, R.I.M., (1988) *Primate societies.* London: Chapman and Hall.

Dunkel, C. S., & Sefcek, J. A. (2009). Eriksonian lifespan theory and life history theory: An integration using the example of identity formation. *Review of General Psychology, 13*(1), 13-23.

Easterbrooks, M., & Lamb, M. (1979). The Relationship between Quality of Infant-Mother Attachment and Infant Competence in Initial Encounters with Peers. *Child Development, 50*(2), 380-387.

Eisenberg, N., Fabes, R., Shepard, S., Guthrie, I., Murphy, B., & Reiser, M. (1999). Parental Reactions to Children's Negative Emotions: Longitudinal Relations to Quality of Children's Social Functioning. *Child Development, 70*(2), 513-534.

El-Sheikh, M., Buckhalt, J., Mize, J., & Acebo, C. (2006). Marital Conflict and Disruption of Children's Sleep. *Child Development, 77*(1), 31-43.

El-Sheikh, M., Kouros, C., Erath, S., Cummings, E., Keller, P., Staton, L., Collins, W. (2009). Marital Conflict and Children's Externalizing Behavior: Interactions between Parasympathetic and Sympathetic Nervous System Activity. *Monographs of the Society for Research in Child Development, 74*(1), I-102.

Erikson, E.H. (1993) *Childhood and Society.* (2nd ed.). New York: Norton.

Erikson, E. H., & Erikson, J.M. (1998) *The Life Cycle Completed.* New York: Norton.

Eysenck, H.J. (1967) *The biological basis of personality.* Springfield: Thomas.

Feminism and Breastfeeding: Rhetoric, Ideology, and the Material Realities of Women's Lives. (2012). In Hausman B., Smith P., & Labbok M. (Eds.), *Beyond Health, Beyond Choice: Breastfeeding Constraints and Realities* (pp. 15-24). Rutgers University Press.

Fernald, A., & Mazzie, C. (1991). Prosody and focus in speech to infants and adults. *Developmental Psychology, 27,* 209-21.

Fewtrell, M. (2011). When to wean? How good is the evidence for six months' exclusive breastfeeding. *BMJ: British Medical Journal,342*(7790), 209-212.

Fillo, J., Simpson, J. A., Rholes, W. S., & Kohn, J. L. (2015). *Dads Journal of Personality and Social Psychology, 108*(2), 298-316.

Flykt, M., Lindblom, J., Punamäki, R.-L., Poikkeus, P., Repokari, L., Unkila-Kallio, L.,… Tulppala, M. (2011). Prenatal expectations in transition to parenthood: Former infertility and family dynamic considerations. *Couple and Family Psychology: Research and Practice, 1*(S), 31-44.

Foss, K. (2018). "That's Not a Beer Bong; It's a Breast Pump!": Representations of Breastfeeding in Prime-Time Fictional Television. In Short A., Palko A., & Irving D. (Eds.), *Breastfeeding and Culture: Discourses and Representation* (pp. 93-111). Bradford: Demeter Press.

Fredman, S. J., Le, Y., Marshall, A. D., Brick, T. R., & Feinberg, M. E. (2017). A dyadic perspective on PTSD symptoms' associations with couple functioning and parenting stress in first-time parents. *Couple and Family Psychology: Research and Practice, 6*(2), 117-132.

Gallegos, M. I., Murphy, S. E., Benner, A. D., Jacobvitz, D. B., & Hazen, N. L. (2017). Marital, parental, and whole-family predictors of toddlers' emotion regulation: The role of parental emotional withdrawal. *Journal of Family Psychology, 31*(3), 294-303.

Galst, J. P. (2018). The elusive connection between stress and infertility: A research review with clinical implications. Journal of Psychotherapy Integration, 28(1), 1-13.

Garbarino, S., Sannita, W. G., & Falkenstein, M. (2017). Inadequate sleeping impairs brain function and aggravates everyday's life: A challenge for human psychophysiology? *Journal of Psychophysiology, 31*(3), 91-93.

Giesbrecht, T., Smeets, T., Leppink, J., Jelicic, M., & Merckelbach, H. (2007). Acute dissociation after 1 night of sleep loss. *Journal of Abnormal Psychology, 116*(3), 599-606.

Gillespie, L., & Hunter, A. (2008). Emotional Flooding—Using Empathy to Help Babies Manage Strong Emotions. *YC Young Children, 63*(5), 46-47.

Givens, D. (1977). INFANTILE REFLEXIVE BEHAVIORS AND NONVERBAL COMMUNICATION. *Sign Language Studies,* (16), 219-236.

Glickstein, M. (2014). Motivation. In *Neuroscience: A Historical Introduction* (pp. 257-270). Cambridge, Massachusetts; London. England: Mit Press.

Goebel, B. L., & Brown, D. R. (1981). Age differences in motivation related to Maslow's need hierarchy. *Developmental Psychology, 17*(6), 809-815.

Goldberg, A. E., Kinkler, L. A., Moyer, A. M., & Weber, E. (2014). Intimate relationship challenges in early parenthood among lesbian, gay, and heterosexual couples adopting via the child welfare system. *Professional Psychology: Research and Practice, 45*(4), 221-230.

Gou, L. H., & Woodin, E. M. (2017). Relationship dissatisfaction as a mediator for the link between attachment insecurity and psychological aggression over the transition to parenthood. *Couple and Family Psychology: Research and Practice, 6*(1), 1-17.

Gómez, R., Bootzin, R., & Nadel, L. (2006). Naps Promote Abstraction in Language-Learning Infants. *Psychological Science,17*(8), 670-674.

Greenfield, E. (2011). Grandparent Involvement and Parenting Stress among Non-married Mothers of Young Children. *Social Service Review, 85*(1), 135-157.

Greenough, W., Black, J., & Wallace, C. (1987). Experience and Brain Development. *Child Development, 58*(3), 539-559.

Grodstein, F., Goldman, M., Ryan, L., & Cramer, D. (1993). Self-Reported Use of Pharmaceuticals and Primary Ovulatory Infertility. *Epidemiology, 4*(2), 151-156.

Grund, A., Fries, S., & Rheinberg, F. (2018). Know your preferences: Self-regulation as need-congruent goal selection. *Review of General Psychology, 22*(4), 437-451.

Gutek, B., Nakamura, C., & Nieva, V. (1981). The Interdependence of Work and Family Roles. *Journal of Occupational Behaviour, 2*(1), 1-16.

Hadley, K. (2009). How Do Parenting Practices Affect Children's Peer Culture? Examining the Intersection of Class and Race. *Race, Gender & Class, 16*(1/2), 6-24.

Hahn, C. S., & DiPietro, J. A. (2001). In vitro fertilization and the family: Quality of parenting, family functioning, and child psychosocial adjustment. *Developmental Psychology, 37*(1), 37-48.

Hale, L., Berger, L. M., LeBourgeois, M. K., & Brooks-Gunn, J. (2011). A longitudinal study of preschoolers' language-based bedtime routines, sleep duration, and well-being. *Journal of Family Psychology, 25*(3), 423-433.

Hall, D. T. and Foster, L. W. (2017). A Psychological Success Cycle And Goal Setting: Goals, Performance, And Attitudes. *Academy of Management Journal, 20*, 2.

Harlow, H. (1958). The Nature of Love. *American Psychologist, 13*, 673-685.

Harrison, Y., & Horne, J. A. (2000). The impact of sleep deprivation on decision-making: A review. *Journal of Experimental Psychology: Applied, 6*(3), 236-249.

Hebbeler, K., & Spiker, D. (2016). Supporting Young Children with Disabilities. *The Future of Children, 26*(2), 185-205.

Held, L., & Rutherford, A. (2012). Can't a mother sing the blues? Postpartum depression and the construction of motherhood in late 20th-century America. *History of Psychology, 15*(2), 107-123.

Hendrick, V. (2003). Treatment Of Postnatal Depression: Effective Interventions Are Available, But The Condition Remains Under-diagnosed. *BMJ: British Medical Journal, 327*(7422), 1003-1004.

Herbst A, et al. (2007). Time between membrane rupture and delivery and septicemia in term neonates. *Obstetrics & Gynecology, 110*, 612.

Herscovitch, J., & Broughton, R. (1981). Performance deficits following short-term partial sleep deprivation and subsequent recovery oversleeping. *Canadian Journal of Psychology/Revue canadienne de psychologie, 35*(4), 309-322.

Hideg, I., Krstic, A., Trau, R. N. C., & Zarina, T. (2018). The unintended consequences of maternity leaves: How agency interventions mitigate the negative effects of longer legislated maternity leaves. *Journal of Applied Psychology, 103*(10), 1155-1164.

Hollander, D. (2004). Postpartum Sexual Problems Are Similar for Depressed and Non-depressed Women, but Prevalence Differs. *Perspectives on Sexual and Reproductive Health, 36*(3), 135-135.

Hostinar, C., Stellern, S., Schaefer, C., Carlson, S., & Gunnar, M. (2012). Associations between early life adversity and executive function in children adopted internationally from orphanages. *Proceedings of the National Academy of Sciences of the United States of America, 109*, 17208-17212.

Jean-Philippe Chaput, Geneviève Leduc, Charles Boyer, Priscilla Bélanger, Allana G. LeBlanc, Michael M. Borghese, & Mark S. Tremblay. (2014). Electronic screens in children's bedrooms and adiposity, physical activity and sleep: Do the number and type of electronic devices matter? *Canadian Journal of Public Health / Revue Canadienne De Santé Publique, 105*(4), E273-E279.

Johnson, M. (2005). Family Roles and Work Values: Processes of Selection and Change. *Journal of Marriage and Family, 67*(2), 352-369.

Jones, E. (2010). Parental relationships and parenting. In Hansen K., Joshi H., & Dex S. (Eds.), *Children of the 21st century (Volume 2): The first five years* (pp. 53-76). Bristol, UK: Bristol University Press.

Kagan, J. (2004). *The long shadow of temperament.* Cambridge, Mass: Harvard University Press.

Kelly, R. J., & El-Sheikh, M. (2011). Marital conflict and children's sleep: Reciprocal relations and socioeconomic effects. *Journal of Family Psychology, 25*(3), 412-422.

Kelly, K.R., Jugovic, H. (2001). Concurrent Validity of the Online Version of the Keirsey Temperament Sorter II. *Journal of Career Assessment, 9*, 49-59.

Keirsey, D. (1998) P*lease Understand Me II: Temperament, Character, Intelligence, 3rd Edition*. Prometheus Nemesis Book Co.

Kime, N. (2008). Children's Eating Behaviours: The Importance of the Family Setting. *Area, 40*(3), 315-322.

Kranz, D., Busch, H., & Niepel, C. (2018). Desires and intentions for fatherhood: A comparison of childless gay and heterosexual men in Germany. *Journal of Family Psychology, 32*(8), 995-1004.

Kris De Welde. (2017). Moving the Needle on Equity and Inclusion. *Humboldt Journal of Social Relations, 39*, 192-211.

KRUK, E. (2013). Sixteen Arguments in Support of Equal Parenting. In *The Equal Parent Presumption: Social Justice in the Legal Determination of Parenting after Divorce* (pp. 98-122). Montreal; Kingston; London; Ithaca: McGill-Queen's University Press.

Kuo, P. X., & Ward, L. M. (2016). Contributions of television use to beliefs about fathers and gendered family roles among first-time expectant parents. *Psychology of Men & Masculinity, 17*(4), 352-362.

Kuo, P. X., Volling, B. L., & Gonzalez, R. (2018). Gender role beliefs, work–family conflict, and father involvement after the birth of a second child. *Psychology of Men & Masculinity, 19*(2), 243-256.

Lamborn, S., Mounts, N., Steinberg, L., & Dornbusch, S. (1991). Patterns of Competence and Adjustment among Adolescents from Authoritative, Authoritarian, Indulgent, and Neglectful Families. *Child Development, 62*(5), 1049-1065.

Lang, S. N., Schoppe-Sullivan, S. J., Kotila, L. E., & Kamp Dush, C. M. (2013). Daily parenting engagement among new mothers and fathers: The role of romantic attachment in dual-earner families. *Journal of Family Psychology, 27*(6), 862-872.

Lavner, J. A., Waterman, J., & Peplau, L. A. (2014). Parent adjustment over time in gay, lesbian, and heterosexual parent families adopting from foster care. *American Journal of Orthopsychiatry, 84*(1), 46-53.

Le, Y., Fredman, S. J., & Feinberg, M. E. (2017). Parenting stress mediates the association between negative affectivity and harsh parenting: A longitudinal dyadic analysis. *Journal of Family Psychology, 31*(6), 679-688.

Le, Y., Fredman, S. J., McDaniel, B. T., Laurenceau, J.-P., & Feinberg, M. E. (2018). Cross-day influences between couple closeness and co-parenting support among new parents. *Journal of Family Psychology.* Advance online publication.

Leerkes, E. M., & Zhou, N. (2018). Maternal sensitivity to distress and attachment outcomes: Interactions with sensitivity to non-distress and infant temperament. *Journal of Family Psychology, 32*(6), 753-761.

Leger, D., Thompson, R., Merritt, J., & Benz, J. (1996). Adult Perception of Emotion Intensity in Human Infant Cries: Effects of Infant Age and Cry Acoustics. *Child Development, 67*(6), 3238-3249.

Leung, P., & Kwan, K. (1998). Parenting Styles, Motivational Orientations, and Self-Perceived Academic Competence: A Meditational Model. *Merrill-Palmer Quarterly, 44*(1), 1-19.

Lewin, R., (1999). *Human evolution.* London: Blackwell Science.

Lewis, M., & Stieben, J. (2004). Emotion Regulation in the Brain: Conceptual Issues and Directions for Developmental Research. *Child Development, 75*(2), 371-376.

Lillard, A. S., Drell, M. B., Richey, E. M., Boguszewski, K., & Smith, E. D. (2015). Further examination of the immediate impact of television on children's executive function. *Developmental Psychology, 51*(6), 792-805.

Lim, J., & Dinges, D. F. (2010). A meta-analysis of the impact of short-term sleep deprivation on cognitive variables. *Psychological Bulletin, 136*(3), 375-389.

Liu, W. M. (2017). White male power and privilege: The relationship between White supremacy and social class. *Journal of Counseling Psychology, 64*(4), 349-358.

Locke, E. A. (1966). The relationship of intentions to level of performance. *Journal of Applied Psychology, 50,* 60-66.

Locke, E. A., & Latham, G. P. (1990). *A theory of goal setting & task performance.* Englewood Cliffs, NJ: Prentice Hall.

Locke, E. A. (1991). Goal theory vs. control theory: Contrasting approaches to understanding work motivation. *Motivation & Emotion, 15,* 9-28.

Locke, A. (2012). Preparing Women to Breastfeed: Teaching Breastfeeding in Prenatal Classes in the United Kingdom. In Smith P., Hausman B., & Labbok M. (Eds.), *Beyond Health, Beyond Choice: Breastfeeding Constraints and Realities* (pp. 110-120). Rutgers University Press.

Lounsbury, M., & Bates, J. (1982). The Cries of Infants of Differing Levels of Perceived Temperamental Difficultness: Acoustic Properties and Effects on Listeners. *Child Development, 53*(3), 677-686.

Loprinzi, P. D., and Davis, R. E. (2016) Secular trends in parent-reported television viewing among children in the United States, 2001–2012. *Child: Care, Health and Development, 42*, 288–291.

Jugovac, D., & Cavallero, C. (2012). Twenty-four hours of total sleep deprivation selectively impairs attentional networks. *Experimental Psychology, 59*(3), 115-123.

Molly, A. (2015). Sleep training at 8 weeks: 'Do you have the guts?'. *The New York Times.* Retrieved from http://www.nytimes.com

McClure, S., Laibson, D., Loewenstein, G., & Cohen, J. (2004). Separate Neural Systems Value Immediate and Delayed Monetary Rewards. *Science, 306*(5695), 503-507.

McDaniel, B. T., & Teti, D. M. (2012). Co-parenting quality during the first three months after birth: The role of infant sleep quality. *Journal of Family Psychology, 26*(6), 886-895.

McIntosh, P. (1988). White Privilege and Male Privilege: A Personal Account of Coming To See Correspondences through Work in Women's Studies. *Working Paper, 189.*

McLeod, J., & Shanahan, M. (1993). Poverty, Parenting, and Children's Mental Health. *American Sociological Review, 58*(3), 351-366.

McHenry, H.M., (1996). Sexual dimorphism in fossil hominids and its sociological implications. In J. Steele and S. Shennan (Eds.), *The archaeology oh human ancestry* (pp.99-109). London: Routledge

McMahon, C. A., Gibson, F., Leslie, G., Cohen, J., & Tennant, C. (2003). Parents of 5-year-old in vitro fertilization children: Psychological adjustment, parenting stress and the influence of subsequent in vitro fertilization treatment. *Journal of Family Psychology, 17*(3), 361-369.

McNeill, D., (2000). *Language and gesture.* Cambridge: Cambridge University Press.

Ma, C. (2018). "I'm MY Breastfeeding Expert": How First-Time Mothers Reclaimed their Power through Breastfeeding. In EINION A. & RINALDI J. (Eds.), *Bearing the Weight of the World: Exploring Maternal Embodiment* (pp. 203-220). Bradford: Demeter Press.

Manchester, J. (2003). Beyond Accommodation: Reconstructing the Insanity Defense to Provide an Adequate Remedy for Postpartum Psychotic Women. *The Journal of Criminal Law and Criminology (1973-), 93*(2/3), 713-752.

Manning, W., Fettro, M., & Lamidi, E. (2014). Child Weil-Being in Same-Sex Parent Families: Review of Research Prepared for American Sociological Association Amicus Brief. *Population Research and Policy Review, 33*(4), 485-502.

Mannering, A., Leve, L., Shaw, D., Neiderhiser, J., Harold, G., Shelton, K.,… Reiss, D. (2011). Longitudinal Associations Between Marital Instability and Child Sleep Problems Across Infancy and Toddlerhood in Adoptive Families. *Child Development, 82*(4), 1252-1266.

Manley, M. H., Goldberg, A. E., & Ross, L. E. (2018). Invisibility and involvement: LGBTQ community connections among plurisexual women during pregnancy and postpartum. *Psychology of Sexual Orientation and Gender Diversity, 5*(2), 169-181.

Marable, M. (1983). Peace and Black Liberation: The Contributions of W.E.B. Du Bois. *Science & Society, 47*(4), 385-405.

Martin, J., Anderson, J. E., Groh, A. M., Waters, T. E. A., Young, E., Johnson, W. F.,… Roisman, G. I. (2018). Maternal sensitivity during the first 3½ years of life predicts electrophysiological responding to and cognitive appraisals of infant crying at midlife. *Developmental Psychology, 54*(10), 1917-1927.

Mäkelä, T. E., Peltola, M. J., Nieminen, P., Paavonen, E. J., Saarenpää-Heikkilä, O., Paunio, T., & Kylliäinen, A. (2018). Nightawakening in infancy: Developmental stability and longitudinal associations with psychomotor development. *Developmental Psychology, 54*(7), 1208-1218.

Mason, M., & Goulden, M. (2004). Marriage and Baby Blues: Redefining Gender Equity in the Academy. *The Annals of the American Academy of Political and Social Science, 596*, 86-103.

Mata, J., Richter, D., Schneider, T., & Hertwig, R. (2018). How cohabitation, marriage, separation, and divorce influence BMI: A prospective panel study. *Health Psychology, 37*(10), 948-958.

Mattanah, J. (2001). Parental Psychological Autonomy and Children's Academic Competence and Behavioral Adjustment in Late Childhood: More Than Just Limit-Setting and Warmth. *Merrill-Palmer Quarterly, 47*(3), 355-376.

Meadow, T., & Stacey, J. (2006). Families. *Contexts, 5*(4), 55-57.

Medina, A. M., Lederhos, C. L., & Lillis, T. A. (2009). Sleep disruption and decline in marital satisfaction across the transition to parenthood. *Families, Systems, & Health, 27*(2), 153-160.

Meezan, W., & Rauch, J. (2005). Gay Marriage, Same-Sex Parenting, and America's Children. *The Future of Children, 15*(2), 97-115.

Milan, S., Snow, S., & Belay, S. (2007). The context of preschool children's sleep: Racial/ethnic differences in sleep locations, routines, and concerns. *Journal of Family Psychology, 21*(1), 20-28.

Miller, G., (2000). Evolution of human music through sexual selection. In N. L. Wallin, B. Merker, and S. Brown (Eds.),*The origins of music* (pp.329-60). Cambridge, MA: Massachusetts Institute of Technology.

Miller, K. F., Arbel, R., Shapiro, L. S., Han, S. C., & Margolin, G. (2018). Does the cortisol awakening response link childhood adversity to adult BMI? *Health Psychology, 37*(6), 526-529.

Minkel, J. D., Banks, S., Htaik, O., Moreta, M. C., Jones, C. W., McGlinchey, E. L.,... Dinges, D. F. (2012). Sleep deprivation and stressors: Evidence for elevated negative affect in response to mild stressors when sleep deprived. *Emotion, 12*(5), 1015-1020.

Morelli, G. A., Rogoff, B., Oppenheim, D., & Goldsmith, D. (1992). Cultural variation in infants' sleeping arrangements: Questions of independence. *Developmental Psychology, 28*(4), 604-613.

Moss, D. (1988). POSTPARTUM PSYCHOSIS DEFENSE: New defensive measure for mothers who kill infants. *ABA Journal,74*(8), 22-22.

Murray, S. L., Seery, M. D., Lamarche, V. M., Kondrak, C., & Gomillion, S. (2018). Implicitly imprinting the past on the present: Automatic partner attitudes and the transition to parenthood. *Journal of Personality and Social Psychology.* Advance online publication.

Murray, S. L., Lamarche, V. M., Gomillion, S., Seery, M. D., & Kondrak, C. (2017). In defense of commitment: The curative power of violated expectations. *Journal of Personality and Social Psychology, 113*(5), 697-729.

Musters, C., McDonald, E., & Jones, I. (2008). Management of Postnatal Depression. *BMJ: British Medical Journal, 337*(7666), 399-403.

Nathoo, T., & Ostry, A. (2014). Promoting Breastfeeding, Solving Social Problems: Exploring State Involvement in Breastfeeding. In Paterson S., Scala F., & Sokolon M. (Eds.), *Fertile Ground: Exploring Reproduction in Canada* (pp. 280-299). McGill-Queen's University Press.

NEANDER, W., & MORSE, J. (1989). Tradition and Change in the Northern Alberta Woodlands Cree: Implications for Infant Feeding Practices. *Canadian Journal of Public Health / Revue Canadienne De Sante'e Publique, 80*(3), 190-194.

Nelson, S. K., Kushlev, K., & Lyubomirsky, S. (2014). The pains and pleasures of parenting: When, why, and how is parenthood associated with more or less well-being? *Psychological Bulletin, 140*(3), 846-895.

Nuttall, A. K., Valentino, K., & Borkowski, J. G. (2012). Maternal history of parentification, maternal warm responsiveness, and children's externalizing behavior. *Journal of Family Psychology, 26*(5), 767-775.

Nuttall, A. K., Valentino, K., Wang, L., Lefever, J. B., & Borkowski, J. G. (2015). Maternal history of parentification and warm responsiveness: The mediating role of knowledge of infant development. *Journal of Family Psychology, 29*(6), 863-872.

Nye, F. (1974). Emerging and Declining Family Roles. *Journal of Marriage and Family, 36*(2), 238-245.

Oliveira, V., Goulart, M., Nobre, J. C., Lucion, M. K., Silveira, P. P., & Bizarro, L. (2017). Emotional interference of baby and adult faces on automatic attention in parenthood. *Psychology & Neuroscience, 10*(2), 144-153.

Onat, G., & Aba, Y. (2015). The Effects of a Healthy Lifestyle and of Anxiety Levels on IVF Outcomes. *African Journal of Reproductive Health / La Revue Africaine De La Santé Reproductive, 19*(4), 92-101.

Ortiz, C., & McCormick, L. (2007). Behavioral parent-training approaches for the treatment of bedtime noncompliance in young children. *Journal of Early and Intensive Behavior Intervention, 4*(2), 511-525.

OSTLER, R., & KRANZ, P. (1976). More Effective Communication Through Understanding Young Children's Nonverbal Behavior. *Young Children, 31*(2), 113-120.

Patrick, G. T. W., & Gilbert, J. A. (1896). Studies from the psychological laboratory of the University of Iowa: On the effects of loss of sleep. *Psychological Review, 3*(5), 469-483.

Paulus, M., Licata, M.,, Gniewosz, B., & Sodian, B. (2018)., The impact of mother-child interaction quality and cognitive abilities on children's self-concept and self-esteem, *Cognitive Development, ,* 48, (42-51).

Perry, C., Quinn, L., & Nelson, J. (2002). Case Study: Birth Plans and Professional Autonomy. *The Hastings Center Report, 32*(2), 12-13.

Peters, H., & Dush, C. (Eds.). (2009). *Marriage and Family: Perspectives and Complexities*. Columbia University Press.

Peterson, B., Newton, C., Rosen, K., & Schulman, R. (2006). Coping Processes of Couples Experiencing Infertility. *Family Relations, 55*(2), 227-239.

Planalp, E. M., Van Hulle, C., Lemery-Chalfant, K., & Goldsmith, H. H. (2017). Genetic and environmental contributions to the development of positive affect in infancy. *Emotion, 17*(3), 412-420.

Plavcan, J. M., & Van Schaik, C. P. (1992). Intrasexual competition and canine dimorphism in anthropoid primates. *American Journal of Physical Anthropology, 87,* 461-77.

Pinquart, M., & Kauser, R. (2018). Do the associations of parenting styles with behavior problems and academic achievement vary by culture? Results from a meta-analysis. *Cultural Diversity and Ethnic Minority Psychology, 24*(1), 75-100.

PIZER, G., WALTERS, K., & MEIER, R. (2007). Bringing Up Baby with Baby Signs: Language Ideologies and Socialization in Hearing Families. *Sign Language Studies, 7*(4), 387-430.

Philbrook, L. E., & Teti, D. M. (2016). Bidirectional associations between bedtime parenting and infant sleep: Parenting quality, parenting practices, and their interaction. *Journal of Family Psychology, 30*(4), 431-441.

Polzella, D. J. (1975). Effects of sleep deprivation on short-term recognition memory. *Journal of Experimental Psychology: Human Learning and Memory, 1*(2), 194-200.

Powell, B., Bolzendahl, C., Geist, C., & Steelman, L. (2010). *Counted Out: Same-Sex Relations and Americans' Definitions of Family*. Russell Sage Foundation.

Power, A., Willmot, H., & Davidson, R. (2011). *Family futures: Childhood and poverty in urban neighbourhoods*. Bristol, UK; Portland, OR, USA: Bristol University Press.

Radunovich, H. L., Smith, S. R., Ontai, L., Hunter, C., & Cannella, R. (2017). The role of partner support in the physical and mental health of poor, rural mothers. *Journal of Rural Mental Health, 41*(4), 237-247.

Rapely, G. (2008). *Baby-led Weaning: Helping Your Baby Love Good Food.* Vermilion Publishing: Great Britain.

Rashley, L. (2005). "Work It out with Your Wife": Gendered Expectations and Parenting Rhetoric Online. *NWSA Journal,17*(1), 58-92.

Rasch, B., & Born, J. (2008). Reactivation and Consolidation of Memory during Sleep. *Current Directions in Psychological Science, 17*(3), 188-192.

Ratcliff, R., & Van Dongen, H. P. A. (2018). The effects of sleep deprivation on item and associative recognition memory. *Journal of Experimental Psychology: Learning, Memory, and Cognition, 44*(2), 193-208.

Reader, J. M., Teti, D. M., & Cleveland, M. J. (2017). Cognitions about infant sleep: Interparental differences, trajectories across the first year, and co-parenting quality. *Journal of Family Psychology, 31*(4), 453-463.

Rettew, D., (2013). *Child Temperament: New Thinking About the Boundary Between Traits and Illness.* New York: Norton Professional Book.

Riskind, R. G., & Tornello, S. L. (2017). Sexual orientation and future parenthood in a 2011–2013 nationally representative United States sample. *Journal of Family Psychology, 31*(6), 792-798.

Riskind, R. G., Patterson, C. J., & Nosek, B. A. (2013). Childless lesbian and gay adults' self-efficacy about achieving parenthood. *Couple and Family Psychology: Research and Practice, 2*(3), 222-235.

Balbernie, R. (2001) Circuits and circumstances: the neurobiological consequences of early relationship experiences and how they shape later behaviour, *Journal of Child Psychotherapy, 27*(3), 237-255.

Robinson, M. A., & Brewster, M. E. (2014). Motivations for fatherhood: Examining internalized heterosexism and gender-role conflict with childless gay and bisexual men. *Psychology of Men & Masculinity, 15*(1), 49-59.

Robinson-Wood, T., Balogun-Mwangi, O., Weber, A., Zeko-Underwood, E., Rawle, S.-A. C., Popat-Jain, A., Cook, E. (2018). "What is it going to be like?": A phenomenological investigation of racial, gendered, and sexual microaggressions among highly educated individuals. Qualitative Psychology. Advance online publication.

Sadeh, A., Flint-Ofir, E., Tirosh, T., & Tikotzky, L. (2007). Infant sleep and parental sleep-related cognitions. *Journal of Family Psychology, 21*(1), 74-87.

Sadeh, A., Keinan, G., & Daon, K. (2004). Effects of stress on sleep: The moderating role of coping style. *Health Psychology, 23*(5), 542-545.

Saxbe, D., Rossin-Slater, M., & Goldenberg, D. (2018). The transition to parenthood as a critical window for adult health. *American Psychologist, 73(9)*, 1190-1200.

Schore, A. (2002). The Neurobiology of Attachment and Early Personality Organization. *Journal of Prenatal & Perinatal Psychology & Health, 16 (3),* 249-263.

Sigillo, A. E., Miller, M. K., & Weiser, D. A. (2012). Attitudes toward nontraditional women using IVF: The importance of political affiliation and religious characteristics. *Psychology of Religion and Spirituality, 4(4),* 249-263.

Sidle, S. (2007). Pain or Gain: Is There a Bright Side to Juggling Work and Family Roles? *Academy of Management Perspectives,21*(4), 80-82.

Siegfried, W. (2014). The Formation and Structure of the Human Psyche

Id, Ego, and Super-Ego – The Dynamic (Libidinal) and Static Unconsciousness, Sublimation, and the Social Dimension of Identity Formation. *Athene Noctua: Undergraduate Philosophy Journal, 2*, 1-3.

Simon, K. A., Tornello, S. L., Farr, R. H., & Bos, H. M. W. (2018). Envisioning future parenthood among bisexual, lesbian, and heterosexual women. *Psychology of Sexual Orientation and Gender Diversity, 5*(2), 253-259.

Schore, A. N. (2001), Effects of a secure attachment relationship on right brain development, affect regulation, and infant mental health. *Infant Mental Health Journal, 22*, 7-66.

Shreffler, K., Tiemeyer, S., Dorius, C., Spierling, T., Greil, A., & McQuillan, J. (2016). Infertility and fertility intentions, desires, and outcomes among US women. *Demographic Research, 35*, 1149-1168.

Simons, R., Lorenz, F., Conger, R., & Wu, C. (1992). Support from Spouse as Mediator and Moderator of the Disruptive Influence of Economic Strain on Parenting. *Child Development, 63*(5), 1282-1301.

Simons, R., Beaman, J., Conger, R., & Chao, W. (1993). Childhood experience, conceptions of parenting, and attitudes of spouse as determinants of parental behavior. *Journal of Marriage and Family, 55*(1), 91-106.

Simons, R., Beaman, J., Conger, R., & Chao, W. (1992). Gender Differences in the Intergenerational Transmission of Parenting Beliefs. *Journal of Marriage and Family, 54*(4), 823-836.

Spera, C. (2005). A Review of the Relationship Among Parenting Practices, Parenting Styles, and Adolescent School Achievement. *Educational Psychology Review, 17*(2), 125-146.

Smith, P., Hausman, B., & Labbok, M. (Eds.). (2012). *Beyond Health, Beyond Choice: Breastfeeding Constraints and Realities*. Rutgers University Press.

SMITH, H. (2005). *Parenting for Primates*. CAMBRIDGE, MASSACHUSETTS; LONDON, ENGLAND: Harvard University Press.

Sokol, Justin T. (2009) "Identity Development Throughout the Lifetime: An Examination of Eriksonian Theory," *Graduate Journal of Counseling Psychology, 1*, 13-27.

Sockol, L. E., & Allred, K. M. (2018). Correlates of symptoms of depression and anxiety among expectant and new fathers. *Psychology of Men & Masculinity, 19*(3), 362-372.

South, S. C., Lim, E., Jarnecke, A. M., & Foli, K. J. (2018). Relationship quality from pre- to post placement in adoptive couples. *Journal of Family Psychology.* Advanced online publication.

Stansbury, K., & Gunnar, M. (1994). Adrenocortical Activity and Emotion Regulation. *Monographs of the Society for Research in Child Development, 59*(2/3), 108-134.

Staton, S. L., Smith, S. S., & Thorpe, K. J. (2015). "Do I really need a nap?": The role of sleep science in informing sleep practices in early childhood education and care settings. *Translational Issues in Psychological Science, 1*(1), 32-44.

Stepan, M. E., Fenn, K. M., & Altmann, E. M. (2018). Effects of sleep deprivation on procedural errors. *Journal of Experimental Psychology: General.* Advance online publication.

Sue, D. W. (2009). Racial microaggressions and worldviews. American Psychologist, 64, 220–221.

Sue, D. W. (2010). *Microaggressions in everyday life: race, gender, and sexual orientation.* Hoboken, NJ: John Wiley & Sons Inc.

Sue, D. W. (2013). Race talk: The psychology of racial dialogues. *American Psychologist, 68*(8), 663-672.

Swartz, E. (2009). Diversity: Gatekeeping Knowledge and Maintaining Inequalities. *Review of Educational Research, 79*(2), 1044-1083.

Sweeney, K. K., Goldberg, A. E., & Garcia, R. L. (2017). Not a "mom thing": Predictors of gatekeeping in same-sex and heterosexual parent families. *Journal of Family Psychology, 31*(5), 521-531.

Syed, M., & Seiffge-Krenke, I. (2013). Personality development from adolescence to emerging adulthood: Linking trajectories of ego development to the family context and identity formation. *Journal of Personality and Social Psychology, 104*(2), 371-384.

Symes, N., Mayo, E., & Laird, E. (2018). Breastfeeding and popular culture: Reflections for policy and practice. In Dowling S., Pontin D., & Boyer K. (Eds.), *Social experiences of breastfeeding: Building bridges between research, policy and practice* (pp. 237-244). Bristol, UK; Chicago, IL, USA: Bristol University Press.

Tanner Stapleton, L., & Bradbury, T. N. (2012). Marital interaction prior to parenthood predicts parent–child interaction 9 years later. *Journal of Family Psychology, 26*(4), 479-487.

Teti, D., & Crosby, B. (2012). Maternal Depressive Symptoms, Dysfunctional Cognitions, and Infant Night Waking: The Role of Maternal Nighttime Behavior. *Child Development, 83*(3), 939-953.

Teti, D. M., Shimizu, M., Crosby, B., & Kim, B.-R. (2016). Sleep arrangements, parent–infant sleep during the first year, and family functioning. *Developmental Psychology, 52*(8), 1169-1181.

Teti, D. M., Kim, B.-R., Mayer, G., & Countermine, M. (2010). Maternal emotional availability at bedtime predicts infant sleep quality. *Journal of Family Psychology, 24*(3), 307-315.

Tikotzky, L., & Sadeh, A. (2009). Maternal Sleep-Related Cognitions and Infant Sleep: A Longitudinal Study from Pregnancy through the 1st Year. *Child Development, 80*(3), 860-874.

The Psychologization of Infertility. (2002). In Van Balen F. & Inhorn M. (Eds.), *Infertility around the Globe: New Thinking on Childlessness, Gender, and Reproductive Technologies* (pp. 79-98). Berkeley; Los Angeles; London: University of California Press.

Trevarthen, C., & Aitken, K. (1994). Brain development, infant communication, and empathy disorders: Intrinsic factors in child mental health. *Development and Psychopathology, 6*(4), 597-633.

Triger, Z. (2013). The Child's Worst Interests: Socio-legal Taboos on Same-Sex Parenting and Their Impact on Children's Well-Being. *Israel Studies Review, 28,*(2), 264-281.

Tripathi, S., & Jha, S. K. (2016). Short-term total sleep deprivation alters delay-conditioned memory in the rat. *Behavioral Neuroscience, 130*(3), 325-335.

Ulbricht, J. A., Ganiban, J. M., Button, T. M. M., Feinberg, M., Reiss, D., & Neiderhiser, J. M. (2013). Marital adjustment as a moderator for genetic and environmental influences on parenting. *Journal of Family Psychology, 27*(1), 42-52.

Walker, M. P., & van der Helm, E. (2009). Overnight therapy? The role of sleep in emotional brain processing. *Psychological Bulletin, 135*(5), 731-748.

Ward, M., & Carlson, E. (1995). Associations among Adult Attachment Representations, Maternal Sensitivity, and Infant-Mother Attachment in a Sample of Adolescent Mothers. *Child Development, 66*(1), 69-79.

Wastell, D., & White, S. (2017). The precarious infant brain. In *Blinded by science: The social implications of epigenetics and neuroscience* (pp. 89-110). Bristol, UK; Chicago, IL, USA: Bristol University Press.

Weigert, A., & Hastings, R. (1977). Identity Loss, Family, and Social Change. *American Journal of Sociology, 82*(6), 1171-1185.

Wendland-Carro, J., Piccinini, C., & Millar, W. (1999). The Role of an Early Intervention on Enhancing the Quality of Mother-Infant Interaction. *Child Development, 70*(3), 713-721.

Welford, A. T. (1978) Mental Work-load as a Function of Demand, Capacity, Strategy and Skill. *Ergonomics, 21*(3), 151-167.

Whitesell, C. J., Crosby, B., Anders, T. F., & Teti, D. M. (2018). Household chaos and family sleep during infants' first year. *Journal of Family Psychology, 32*(5), 622-631.

Wilfred H. O. Schmidt, & Hore, T. (1970). Some Nonverbal Aspects of Communication between Mother and Preschool Child. *Child Development, 41*(3), 889-896.

Winston, C. N., Maher, H., & Easvaradoss, V. (2017). Needs and values: An exploration. *The Humanistic Psychologist, 45*(3), 295-311.

Witeck, B. (2014). Cultural change in acceptance of LGBT people: Lessons from social marketing. *American Journal of Orthopsychiatry, 84*(1), 19-22.

Wolf, J. (2011). *Is Breast Best?: Taking on the Breastfeeding Experts and the New High Stakes of Motherhood.* New York; London: NYU Press.

Workman, J. L., Barha, C. K., & Galea, L. A. M. (2012). Endocrine substrates of cognitive and affective changes during pregnancy and postpartum. *Behavioral Neuroscience, 126*(1), 54-72.

Wright, J. C., Huston, A. C., Ross, R. P., Calvert, S. L., Rolandelli, D., Weeks, L. A.,… Potts, R. (1984). Pace and continuity of television programs:

Effects on children's attention and comprehension. *Developmental Psychology, 20*(4), 653-666.

Wrzus, C., Wagner, G. G., & Riediger, M. (2014). Feeling good when sleeping in? Day-to-day associations between sleep duration and affective well-being differ from youth to old age. *Emotion, 14*(3), 624-628.

Wrzus, C., Hänel, M., Wagner, J., & Neyer, F. J. (2013). Social network changes and life events across the life span: A meta-analysis. *Psychological Bulletin, 139*(1), 53-80.

Yan, J., Olsavsky, A., Schoppe-Sullivan, S. J., & Kamp Dush, C. M. (2018). Co-parenting in the family of origin and new parents' couple relationship functioning. *Journal of Family Psychology, 32*(2), 206-216.

Vertsberger, D., & Knafo-Noam, A. (2018). Mothers' and fathers' parenting and longitudinal associations with children's observed distress to limitations: From pregnancy to toddlerhood. *Developmental Psychology, 55*(1), 123-134.

Viala, E. S. (2011). Contemporary family life: A joint venture with contradictions. *Nordic Psychology, 63*(2), 68-87.

Zelazo, P., Müller, U., Frye, D., Marcovitch, S., Argitis, G., Boseovski, J.,... Carlson, S. (2003). The Development of Executive Function in Early Childhood. *Monographs of the Society for Research in Child Development, 68*(3), I-151.

Zeskind, P. (1983). Cross-Cultural Differences in Maternal Perceptions of Cries of Low- and High-Risk Infants. *Child Development, 54*(5), 1119-1128.

Zhou, N., Cao, H., & Leerkes, E. M. (2017). Interparental conflict and infants' behavior problems: The mediating role of maternal sensitivity. *Journal of Family Psychology, 31*(4), 464-474.

Zahavi, A., (1975). Mate selection: a selection of handicap. *Journal of Theoretical Biology, 53,* 205-214.

Zvara, B. J., Macfie, J., Cox, M., Mills-Koonce, R., & The Family Life Project Key Investigators. (2018). Mother–child role confusion, child adjustment problems, and the moderating roles of child temperament and sex. *Developmental Psychology, 54*(10), 1891-1903.

CPSIA information can be obtained
at www.ICGtesting.com
Printed in the USA
FSHW020907120819
60950FS